Reverse Sarcopenia

An Easy-to-Follow Program to Keep Muscles Strong and Youthful While Reducing Your Risk of Developing Dementia

Dr. Joseph Tieri

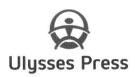

Ulysses Press

Published in the United States by:
Ulysses Press
P.O. Box 3440
Berkeley, CA 94703
www.ulyssespress.com

ISBN13: 978-1-61243-909-9
Library of Congress Control Number 2018967985

Printed in Canada by Marquis Book Printing
10 9 8 7 6 5 4 3 2 1

Acquisitions editor: Bridget Thoreson
Managing editor: Claire Chun
Editors: Lily Chou, Lauren Harrison
Proofreader: Barbara Schultz
Indexer: Sayre Van Young
Front cover design: what!design @ whatweb.com
Photos: © Rapt Productions except cover © kurhan/shutterstock.com; page 10 © Viktoriia Hnatiuk/shutterstock.com, page 25 © Halfpoint/shutterstock.com, page 53 © wavebreakmedia/shutterstock.com, page 55 © Dmytro Zinkevych/shutterstock.com, page 58 © Ken stocker/shutterstock.com, page 103 © Syda Productions/shutterstock.com
Production: Jake Flaherty
Models: Alex Lewin, Kym Sterner

Please note: This book has been written and published strictly for informational purposes, and in no way should be used as a substitute for consultation with healthcare professionals. You should not consider educational material herein to be the practice of medicine or to replace consultation with a physician or other medical practitioner. The author and publisher are providing you with information in this work so that you can have the knowledge and can choose, at your own risk, to act on that knowledge. The author and publisher also urge all readers to be aware of their health status and to consult healthcare professionals before beginning any health program.

For my loving wife, Janice, and my adorable and precious daughters, Lexi and Madie.

Contents

Introduction **7**

Prevalence 8

History 8

Patient Experiences with Weakness 9

Just Being Active Isn't Enough 9

Challenge Your Muscles 10

How to Use This Book 11

No Greater Mission 12

CHAPTER 1

What Is Sarcopenia? **13**

Types of Sarcopenia 14

Causes of Sarcopenia 15

Consequences of Sarcopenia 17

CHAPTER 2

Treating Sarcopenia:
Progressive Resistance Exercises **24**

Osteoporosis and PRE 25

Increasing Strength and Power with PRE 26

The Elderly and PRE 27

Are You Ever Too Sick? 27

Is It Ever Too Late? 28

Do the Benefits Last? 28

Weight and PRE 29

CHAPTER 3

How to Strengthen Muscles **30**

Safety First 30

Proper Form 31

Warming Up and Dynamic Stretches 32

Cooling Down and Static Stretches 43

CHAPTER 4

The Program *52*

Exercises 54
Intensity 55
Repetitions 56
Velocity 56
Sets 56

Rest 57
Frequency 57
Varying Your Routine 57
Tools and Equipment 58

CHAPTER 5

The Exercises *60*

Overhead Press with Weights 62
Overhead Press with Resistance Tube 63
Tennis Backhand with Weights 64
Tennis Backhand with Resistance Tube 65
Tennis Forehand with Weights 66
Tennis Forehand with Resistance Tube 67
Thumbs Up with Weights 68
Thumbs Up with Resistance Tube 69
Chest Press with Weights 70
Standing Chest Press with Resistance Tube 71
Chest Fly with Weights 72
Chest Fly with Resistance Tube 73
Reverse Fly with Weights 74
Seated Row with Resistance Tube 75
Single-Arm Row with Weights 76
Biceps Curl with Weights 77
Biceps Curl with Resistance Tube 78
Bent-Over Triceps Kick-Backs with Weights 79

Standing Triceps Kick-Backs
with Resistance Tubes 80
Curl-Up with Weights 81
Trunk Rotation with Resistance Tube 82
Bird Dog with Weights 83
Prone Extension with Weights 84
Quad Setting 87
Seated Leg Raise with Weights 88
Leg Press with Resistance Tube 89
Standing Leg Curl with Weights 90
Prone Leg Curl with Resistance Tube 91
Chair Squat with Weights 92
Chair Squat with Resistance Tube 93
Squat with Weights 94
Squat with Resistance Tube 95
Seated Leg Extension with Weights 96
Seated Leg Extension with Resistance Tube 97
Heel Raise with Weights 98
Heel Raise with Resistance Tube 99

CHAPTER 6

Sarcopenia and Diet...........................100

Older Adults and Protein Deficits................100

How Much More Protein Should You Eat?.........102

Types and Timing of Proteins...................105

Dietary Recommendations and Tips.............106

Protein Supplementation......................106

Other Supplements............................109

CHAPTER 7

F-A-C-S Process: Sarcopenia Self-Tests............111

Find..111

Assess......................................112

Confirm.....................................114

Severity....................................115

Afterword....................................117

Notes..118

Bibliography.................................120

Index..123

Acknowledgments.............................127

About the Author.............................128

Introduction

"…[sarcopenia] is an independent predictor of all-cause mortality and cognitive impairment, increasing the chances of institutionalization later in life."

—Alex Han and Steven L. Bokshan, et al., in the *Journal of Clinical Medicine*

Believe it or not, by the time you reach the ripe young age of 50, your muscles—which have already been getting weaker for more than a decade—also begin to thin and can lose up to 1 percent of their strength every year. This age-related muscle loss and weakness is called sarcopenia. The disease, along with its consequences, is one of the hottest topics in medicine.

Studies are now revealing that these age-related changes in the muscles create and accompany many more health problems than previously thought, including balance issues that lead to falls, osteoporosis, fractures, and an increased incidence of dementia. The abnormalities that occur in sarcopenia are accompanied by other physiologic changes, resulting in a host of additional medical illnesses, post-surgical complications, and, at a certain point, an increased risk of dying from all conditions!

Fortunately, new information is emerging about strategies to combat the disease. The most important is a simple form of exercise called progressive resistance. While it's more popular among younger gym-goers, progressive resistance exercise (PRE) is well-tolerated and extremely beneficial to adults, even very elderly and frail people. PRE not only slows the progression of sarcopenia, but also reverses and prevents it. Nutritional interventions, especially adequate protein intake, are also showing promise in combating sarcopenia.

Simply put, modern science is learning just how common and debilitating aging muscles can be on the quality and quantity of life, and how effective the right interventions are to keep them strong and healthy. With a little effort, the ability to maintain—or return to—a healthier state, keep physical function and mental capacity intact, and live independently long into your senior years can be a reality. Without it, those things are in serious jeopardy.

Prevalence

Sarcopenia is a widespread public health problem. Though estimates vary, approximately a quarter of people in their 60s already have substantial muscle loss and signs of weakness, and once into their 70s, more than 40 percent of people will have sarcopenia. The problem currently affects more than 50 million older men and women worldwide, and that number is expected to surge to 500 million adults in the next few decades. It's also a costly problem, with more than $20 billion spent each year in the United States on the consequences of the disease.

It begins as early as in one's late 30s. The loss of strength and power happens slowly, declining about 3 to 5 percent per decade. It accelerates to 5 to 10 percent loss per decade as adults reach their 50s, 10 to 15 percent during their 60s, and by the time older adults advance into their 70s, a staggering 25 to 40 percent loss of strength and a 15 percent loss of muscle mass per decade can occur. All totaled, sarcopenia can add up to more than 30 percent muscle loss over a lifetime.

History

The weakness that accompanies aging is nothing new. Marcus Tullius Cicero, a Roman statesman and philosopher, wrote about it in a treatise on old age in 44 B.C. While many lamented the decay of old age, Cicero realized that much could be done about it, advising that it was our duty to "fight against it as we would fight against disease; to adopt a regimen of health; to practice moderate exercise." And while Cicero was right that it is our duty to fight the symptoms of old age, our understanding of this ancient condition has only recently grown—better equipping us for the battle!

While officially coined in 1989, the term "sarcopenia"—from the Greek for "poverty of the flesh"— has newly achieved some uniform diagnostic consensus. Many experts now agree that sarcopenia should include both the signs of age-related muscle loss as well as the symptoms of getting weaker—of functional decline. This collective agreement has resulted in a flurry of new research just in the past decade. While challenges still exist in accurately diagnosing individuals, and there is still a lot to learn in tailoring interventions, the wealth of new information has better defined the condition and brought forth new solutions.

Patient Experiences with Weakness

I frequently observe this in my office: My 50-year-old patients are a little slow to get up from the chair; the 60-year-olds use their arms as they muster more effort to get their legs under them when they rise; and my 70- and 80-year-olds make slight grunting sounds and struggle to gain their balance, slow and unsteady as they begin to walk.

Difficulty getting up from a chair is the tip of the iceberg. My older patients also report problems getting out of cars and climbing stairs, lifting grandchildren and grocery bags, and opening windows and jars. These inconveniences together compromise the ability to perform activities of daily living, or ADLs. Along with the cognitive decline associated with sarcopenia, more and more assistance becomes necessary, and, to the dismay of patients and families alike, independent living is easily lost and nursing home admissions often follow.

Like many physicians, I used to think this weakness was unavoidable—just a normal part of the aging process. And yet, through my clinical experience treating older patients, I have come to know that many of the chronic muscle and joint problems—also believed to be an inevitable aspect of aging—can often be reversed and prevented. Fortunately, the same is true with muscle loss and weakness. Unfortunately, most adults are not doing nearly enough to get stronger and prevent sarcopenia, even those that lead active lives.

Just Being Active Isn't Enough

When I ask patients if they exercise, they frequently respond by saying such things as, "No, but I never sit down," or "I don't have to, I go up and down my stairs all day long." Don't be fooled. While leading an active lifestyle is important, just being active alone will not in itself make you stronger or more fit—it will only allow you to become weaker more slowly. Why? Because the body is smart and conserves energy whenever it can.

If you can already accomplish the task—go up and down the stairs, walk around the block, bike around the neighborhood, or even jog around the track—the body won't devote a lot of resources to the muscles involved. It doesn't have to. Studies of healthy seniors who accurately report lifestyles complete with moderate to vigorous physical activity levels show that their strength level is far from maximal.

Challenge Your Muscles

Of course, if you're out of shape, adopting a more active lifestyle will have a positive effect on the muscles initially, but it will only get you so far. This is also true when it comes to aerobic fitness and its effects on the cardiovascular system and is what prompted me to write my last book, *Staying Young with Interval Training: The Revolutionary HIIT Approach to Getting Fit, Living Healthy, and Keeping Muscles Young.* Research on aerobic training has also demonstrated that after some initial gains, unless you challenge the cardiovascular system, push it to its limits if only for a brief interval, it won't provide the resources to become more fit.

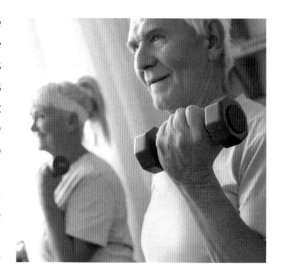

To heed Cicero's advice and effectively battle the health problems that come with aging, to get stronger and more fit, you need to do specific exercises—or more precisely, a specific *way* of exercising. The key is to engage the muscles with enough weight or resistance so that they become tired—at a certain point unable to continue while maintaining proper form. And we need to keep challenging them as they get stronger. As mentioned before, this is what's known as progressive resistance exercise (PRE), and it's a very effective—and ultimately enjoyable—way to stave off frailty and dementia and become stronger and healthier.

Additionally, science is also finding out that nutritional factors play an important role in creating and combating sarcopenia. Not only do older adults often consume inadequate amounts of protein, but also the aging body has challenges absorbing and utilizing proteins and other nutrients. Especially when combined with exercise, nutritional support has been shown to assist the body in building muscle.

How to Use This Book

I recommend you read the first five chapters of this book in succession. Chapter 1 will give you a thorough understanding of what sarcopenia is and, most importantly, its causes and consequences. Unless you recognize how serious sarcopenia is, you may miss your opportunity to prevent or reverse it. Studies have shown that most people who claim not to have enough time (the biggest reason given) to exercise aren't making it a priority because they don't have a big enough reason why they should.

Chapter 2 details numerous studies that demonstrate just how progressive resistance exercise quickly creates strength among people of differing ages and health levels and maintains those benefits for years.

People of all fitness levels should read Chapter 3. This chapter contains important information about exercising safely, plus dynamic stretches for warming up and static stretches for cooling down—both necessary to avoid injury and setbacks.

Chapter 4 describes an overall fitness program for optimal health and, based on the latest research and recommendations, contains specific information on exercise training. The appropriate level of intensity, the ideal number of repetitions and sets, and the amount of rest needed is all discussed in detail to tailor the program to your fitness level and goals. Different training tools and gear options are also discussed.

The potentially life-changing material is found in Chapter 5, which describes more than 35 resistance training exercises using dumbbells, resistance bands, and ankle weights—the most important weapons to defeat sarcopenia and live a life of strength and ability. When you're ready, go for it!

Though especially important for seniors, I recommend everyone read Chapter 6 for vital information regarding nutrition to support your strength regimen and prevent the muscle loss of the senior years. Combined with PRE, it is the cornerstone of sarcopenia treatment.

Finally, to test yourself, or assess an older parent or loved one, I recommend you flip to Chapter 7, which offers a self-assessment questionnaire and several easy-to-do physical tests. These tests are effective for determining whether sarcopenia is present or to get baseline measurement for comparison later. They are also great tools for healthcare practitioners wanting to add sarcopenia testing for their older patients.

No Greater Mission

Millions of Americans will soon become weaker, frailer, and mentally challenged as they reach what should be their retirement or golden years, compromising their ability to live independently and enjoy life fully. There's no doubt about it, sarcopenia is as good a predictor of chronic illness and disease, dementia, and death as it gets.

Fortunately, it doesn't have to happen to you. While some minor muscle loss is inevitable, the absolute amount as well as the rate of loss is, in most instances, under our control. Take dental hygiene: The need for a regular routine of care for a healthy mouth (brushing, flossing, and dental check-ups) is similar to the need of care for the rest of our body—the muscles and joints. If you're like me, you might have noticed that your level of commitment to your teeth and gums has grown as you've aged, with dental cleaning devices taking over more and more counter and drawer space. Like it or not, our bodies also require an increased level of commitment—and tools—to care for them as we age. Ignore it, and you suffer the consequences.

The founding father of fitness himself, Jack LaLanne, is a great example of someone who successfully fought the aging process. Jack finally succumbed to illness at the ripe old age of 96, dying at home, surrounded by loved ones. By all accounts, he exercised to the very end and lived a high-quality, independent life. And believe it or not, Jack claimed not to love exercise. He did, however, understand its importance and the obstacles to it. As Jack himself put it:

"I've only got one enemy: Jack LaLanne…I usually hit the gym around 5 or 6 in the morning. To leave a hot bath, leave a hot woman, go into a cold gym takes a lot of discipline, boy, I'll tell ya…I never liked to exercise, but I like results."

Jack LaLanne had a commitment to health that most will never approximate. When he was 70, Jack towed 70 boats on a 2½-hour, one-mile-long swim. Fortunately, science is showing that significant benefits can be achieved with a lot less Herculean effort. Jack also realized this and advised: "Be yourself…. Find the time three or four days a week to get the blood flowing and the muscles working."

It may take a shift in your outlook or in your attitude toward exercise and the aging process to get out of your own way—to embrace health and fitness. There is no greater mission in life than to understand the importance of waging war against becoming frail and weak—from developing sarcopenia. Once you embrace resistance training and the other tools in this book to get stronger and healthier, your investment in yourself will never have been more worth it. Life goes by fast. We only get one chance, so don't regret not making the most of it. You need a strong body and mind to do so. If you're ready, read on.

CHAPTER 1

What Is Sarcopenia?

"…practitioners have ever-increasing possibilities for preventing, delaying, treating, and sometimes even reversing sarcopenia by way of early and effective interventions."

—European Working Group on Sarcopenia in Older People (EWGSOP)

Until recently, no reliable definition of sarcopenia was universally accepted. With the expansion of research and clinical studies in the past decade, updates to definitions, diagnostic tools, and treatment options were necessary. One of the leading authorities on sarcopenia, the European Working Group on Sarcopenia in Older People (EWGSOP), met for a second time in 2018 to update the healthcare community about sarcopenia. An additional goal of the meeting was to increase awareness of sarcopenia, a devastating yet often overlooked and undertreated disease.

One of the most significant changes that the EWGSOP recommended was to classify sarcopenia as a muscle disease—a failure of muscle to function properly—because of changes accrued over a lifetime. The key components of this muscle disease are the progressive loss of muscle strength (think of this as difficulty lifting your grandchild) and loss of power (think of this as difficulty righting yourself after you trip). Gone from this classification is the overemphasis placed on the decrease in muscle size, or mass, because it is difficult to measure muscle size in a clinical setting, and because the loss of muscle size compared to muscle strength does not always correlate equally.

Some of the group's updated findings include:

> While sarcopenia is still associated with aging, it is now recognized to start earlier than previously thought.

> Sarcopenia has other contributing causes in addition to aging.

> The definition of sarcopenia includes the concept of muscle failure, with the strength of the muscle taking prominence over its size.

> Low muscle quality is also a factor.

> The characteristic of poor physical performance—a criteria related to movement—has been added to identify severe sarcopenia.

EWGSOP's operational diagnosis of sarcopenia is not a major departure: "…a progressive and generalized skeletal muscle disorder that is associated with increased likelihood of adverse outcomes including falls, fractures, physical disability, and mortality." And it's probable when low muscle strength is present.

While sarcopenia is a serious disorder associated with major disabilities, the group reports that sarcopenia can be treated and, in some cases, actually reversed!

Types of Sarcopenia

Primary and Secondary Sarcopenia

Primary sarcopenia exists when age is the only factor—no other medical issues or causes are known. Sarcopenia is secondary when factors other than age are present that may play a role in the muscles' decline. Examples of secondary sarcopenia include those that result from joint problems leading to immobility, and from the muscle wasting that sometimes accompanies cancer.

Acute and Chronic Sarcopenia

The difference between acute and chronic sarcopenia is how long the disease has been present. Acute cases have been present for less than six months. This can be from temporary conditions such as being laid-up because of a recent illness, injury, or surgery. Without intervention, a rapid decline in strength and function can occur. A chronic classification is when the condition has been present for six months or more and is often the result of a sedentary lifestyle or permanent disability. Chronic illnesses and progressive conditions often coexist, making sarcopenia more intractable.

These classifications are important to better define what causes the condition, establish appropriate treatment options, and to emphasize that sarcopenia does not have to be a lifetime diagnosis. They underscore the need to monitor the condition, intervene to remove secondary causes, and provide treatment options in acute cases to prevent them from becoming chronic (for example, a focus on upper-body strengthening in the months following a knee or hip replacement).

Sarcopenic Obesity, aka Skinny-Fat

Sarcopenic obesity (SO), sometimes referred to as skinny-fat, or fat-frail, is a special condition where the reduced muscle mass and strength of sarcopenia is present in an overweight body. SO is characterized by excess visceral fat (the type that surrounds the midsection and abdominal organs) as opposed to subcutaneous fat (fat under the skin). A sarcopenic obese body can mask underlying muscle loss, and someone with SO can have the appearance of an individual with a normal weight. While not a new phenomenon, skinny-fat is fast becoming more prevalent due to the growing trends of a sedentary lifestyle and poor dietary choices upon an aging society.

Though much is still to be learned, it appears that obesity compounds the problems associated with sarcopenia, increasing fat infiltration into lean muscle, and worsening systemic inflammation. As serious and damaging as sarcopenia is, it's even worse for older obese people. A major concern is the increased likelihood of cognitive loss—including problems with memory, orientation, and self-control issues—associated with SO. Additionally, more than either condition alone, SO is associated with the poorest performance on executive function tests. Executive function is the ability to analyze, plan, organize, and follow through on tasks. Fortunately, resistance training has been shown to enhance older individuals' executive cognitive function.

SO also leads to an increased risk of frailty and disability, morbidity, and mortality. And for the subset of the SO population that is also saddled with osteoporosis—newly termed osteosarcopenic obesity (OSO)—problems that are greater than those associated with each of the individual disorders frequently occur.

Causes of Sarcopenia

The mechanisms that lead to sarcopenia are complex and our understanding is still evolving. What is clear, however, is that multiple processes—cellular, hormonal, metabolic, and molecular—are at play, impairing the skeletal muscles. Like what causes aging bones to become thin (osteopenia), the result of this complex activity is that the balance between the building up of body tissue—in this case skeletal muscle—and the breaking down, leans toward breakdown as we age. Some of the mechanisms leading to sarcopenia include:

> Decreased capacity of the muscle to repair itself, a result of fewer satellite cells (cells that have a role in repairing muscles), especially type 2a fibers.

> Diminished sensitivity to insulin, or a reduced secretion of insulin.

> Reduced levels of androgens, estrogens, and growth hormones.

> Difficulty absorbing and utilizing dietary proteins.

> Increased myostatin (or GDF-8), a protein that has a negative effect on muscle growth.

> Reduced tissue oxygenation.

> Reduced concentrations of myosin, a protein instrumental in muscle contraction; its reduction is exacerbated by decreased physical activity.

> Age-related chronic inflammation.

> Possible genetic factors.

On the surface, sarcopenia is associated with thinning and atrophying muscles—a diminished quantity of muscle. Digging deeper, changes to the architecture of the muscle itself can be observed, diminishing its quality. These changes, seen in and around the muscle fibers as well as in the nervous system that influences them, include:

> Fatty infiltration around and between muscle fibers.

> Decrease of type 2a muscle fibers—fast contraction, power-producing, fatigue-resistant fibers.

> Loss of mitochondria—the powerhouses of the cells.

> Reduction in the number of motor units, which often work in groups to coordinate muscle contractions.

> Neuromuscular junction remodeling—changes in the chemical synapses that signal muscles to contract.

The end results are muscle fibrosis, tendon stiffness, a loss of contractility, and a lower capacity to generate force, creating slower, weaker, and less powerful muscles that are less able to right themselves at times of instability—the hallmarks of sarcopenia.

Fortunately, exercise training has been shown to not only have a positive impact on the single fiber and whole muscle levels, but also can slow or reverse some of the other systemic challenges to the body—including age-related inflammation.

While the deleterious impact of sarcopenia on muscles is central to the suffering that results, and is where the treatment will largely be focused, as we've begun to discover, the consequences of the disease reach far beyond the soft tissues.

Consequences of Sarcopenia

The list of problems that sarcopenia is associated with is long and growing. From mental to physical, they are wide-ranging and vary from mild to serious. Perhaps the most distressing consequence of sarcopenia for patients and families alike is when the level of functioning declines to the point that an elderly person loses their independence and must be removed from their home.

You may be surprised to learn that leg strength is one of the most important factors to the body's continued ability to function well and independently. A July 2018 study of older women published in *PLOS One* shows that leg muscle power is even more important in combating the functional decline associated with sarcopenia than aerobic capacity, physical activity level, or even age. That's right: The relative power of your leg muscles is a better indicator of your ability to walk, climb stairs, and perform other activities of daily living (ADLs) like get dressed, do housework, shop, and cook a meal, than how fit or old you are. Assuming you're both seniors, you could be older and less physically active than your neighbor, but because you spend a couple days a week resistance-training your legs, you're in functionally better shape. And here's some amazing news: If you're a man or a woman over the age of 70, your stronger legs decrease your risk of dying from all causes over the next six years (and possibly longer than that).

It may sound startling that the presence of sarcopenia could have such an impact on your very survival. The reason is that the quality and quantity of skeletal muscle has a much wider effect on the health of the human body than just its ability to remain strong and balanced. When you consider that skeletal muscle makes up close to half of an adult's lean body mass, and that skeletal muscle is the body's main organ system for the metabolism of blood sugar after a meal, its significance becomes clear. As muscle cells diminish and become of poorer quality, insulin sensitivity decreases, increasing the likelihood of diabetes and all the problems associated with it—including cardiovascular disease.

Following is a list of some of the specific medical and surgical impacts sarcopenia can have based on a review of thousands of available studies. In some cases, sarcopenia causes these problems; in others, its presence makes them worse.

Cognitive Disorders and Depression

According to the Centers for Disease Control and Prevention (CDC), more than 16 million people in the United States are currently experiencing cognitive impairment, with a dramatic increase expected as more Americans reach their senior years. Sarcopenia has been shown to be significantly associated with cognitive disorders; a 2015 study by Magdalena Tolea and James Galvin in *Clinical Interventions in Aging* showed that people with sarcopenia are six times more likely to have cognitive impairment.

Cognitive impairment ranges from mild to severe. Mild impairments include memory problems, trouble learning new things, and hesitating when making simple decisions. Most people are not aware of their mild impairments, and generally have no problem performing their ADLs. Severe impairment—including dementia and Alzheimer's disease—often includes difficulty communicating, more serious confusion, and lack of understanding, all of which pose a risk to the individual if living alone.

Sarcopenia is also significantly associated with depression. Depression is one of the most prevalent mental disorders in older adults. It's a debilitating disorder characterized by sadness, low self-esteem, and a loss of joy and interest in hobbies and social gatherings. Effects range from more mild—poor sleep, a lack of interest in eating, and concentration problems—to more severe disability and an increased risk of death.

Now here's the good news: Not only can resistance training improve executive cognitive dysfunction, but also debilitating conditions like dementia and depression—devastating and costly to patients and families alike—may find a treatment route through exercise.

Tolea and Galvin write: "Given the success reported for physical activity interventions in improving physical and cognitive performance, even among individuals with sarcopenia, whether working by improving strength via increasing muscle mass or through other pathways, such interventions have the potential to delay development of physical disability and dementia, and therefore address an important public health concern."

And as a 2018 study concluded, "a healthy lifestyle consisting of good nutrition and physical activity/fitness should be promoted as a means to prevent cognitive impairment and/or depression symptoms as well as sarcopenia with normal aging."

Osteoporosis, Bone Fractures, and Bone Disease

Sometimes referred to as the twin conditions of aging, sarcopenia and osteopenia are becoming more common as the country ages. According to the International Osteoporosis Foundation, osteoporosis affects approximately 30 percent of all post-menopausal women in the United States. At least 40 percent of those women, and up to 30 percent of men, will suffer one or more fractures.

While they are separate disorders, sarcopenia is an independent risk factor for osteoporosis. A study examining 600 community residents looked at the relationship between sarcopenia and bone mineral density (BMD), and concluded, "The risk of low BMD increased significantly with sarcopenia."

Sarcopenia is something of a double-edged sword when it comes to causing fractures. On one hand, it leads to lower BMD and weakens bone. And on the other hand, the muscle weakness and loss of power leads to balance issues and falls. Each year, about a third of people over age 65 will experience a fall, setting the stage to fracture bone.

Consider a 2015 report from the annual meeting of the American Society for Bone and Mineral Research, which found that using criteria proposed by the EWGSOP, people with sarcopenia had a significantly greater risk (2.3 times higher) of having a low-trauma fracture from a fall, such as a broken hip, collarbone, leg, arm, or wrist, within three years.

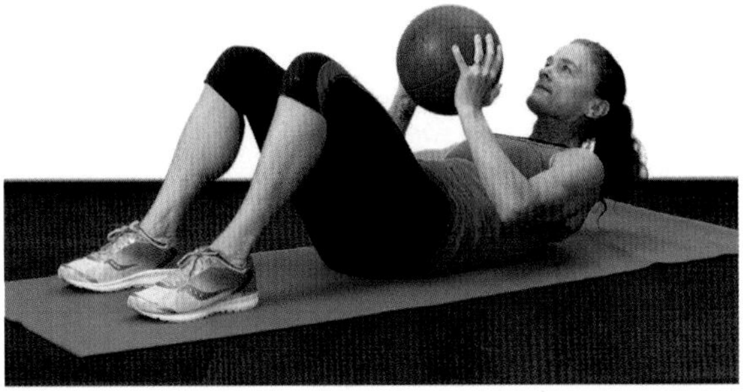

Another study published in *Geriatric Gerontology International* looked for the presence of sarcopenia in 357 patients immediately after suffering a hip fracture, compared to 2,511 patients from the same healthcare facility who hadn't had a hip fracture. The authors concluded, "This study showed a higher prevalence of sarcopenia and more reduced leg muscle mass in patients after a hip fracture than in the out-patient clinic who did not have hip fractures. The results imply sarcopenia can be a risk factor for a hip fracture."

This is serious business, as more than one in four people aged 65 or older die within a year following a hip fracture. This is a death rate that is three times greater than the general population.

In addition to the findings discussed here regarding osteoporosis, a review of the research reveals that sarcopenia is associated with an increased prevalence of multiple osteoporotic vertebral fractures in women, and sarcopenic obese patients have an increased rate of developing knee osteoarthritis (OA).

Muscle and bone are intimately connected and intertwined in the human body, and both need to be stressed or they grow weaker. Not surprisingly, sarcopenia and osteoporosis share common causes, including decreased sensitivity to anabolic hormones, systemic inflammation, and a sedentary lifestyle. Fortunately, the PRE treatments outlined in this book can successfully address both conditions at the same time.

Diabetes

According to the CDC, more than 100 million people in the United States are either diabetic or prediabetic. The prediabetic condition, present in about one of three Americans, is a disorder of higher-than-normal blood sugar levels, but not yet to the level of diabetes. While 90 percent of people with this condition are mostly unaware that they have it, without intervention, 5 to 10 percent of them will progress to type-2 diabetes each year, dramatically increasing their risk for heart attacks and strokes, and kidney, eye, and nerve damage.

A key defect in diabetes and prediabetes is insulin resistance—the refusal of the body's tissue to absorb blood sugar in response to the actions of insulin. The body's abundant skeletal muscle uses the majority of the blood sugar after a meal. Losing lean skeletal muscle and gaining fat cells (along with other changes observed in sarcopenia) can easily create, or exacerbate, insulin resistance. Patients with sarcopenia have been reported to have higher HbA1c levels—a measure of the average blood sugar level over the past two to three months—and be at risk for developing type-2 diabetes with all its associated medical problems.

Fortunately, studies show that physical activity boosts the effects of insulin both to reduce the onset of diabetes and to synthesize muscle protein. Conversely, little to no exercise impairs insulin's ability to do its job.

Cardiovascular Disease

According to an April 2018 sarcopenia research literature review in the *Journal of Clinical Medicine*, people with sarcopenia are more frequently hypertensive, a well-documented condition that increases the risk of cardiovascular disease. Other sobering findings:

> Sarcopenic obese people have increased LDLs (the "bad" cholesterol) and decreased HDLs (the "good" cholesterol).

> People with sarcopenia have reduced left ventricular ejection fraction, which is the amount of blood the heart pumps out (lower numbers signify heart failure).

> There is a higher mortality rate in sarcopenic patients with chronic heart failure.

A 2016 study conducted at the University of California, Los Angeles, Health Sciences department examined data involving 6,451 patients with cardiovascular disease. Those patients who had the highest muscle mass with low fat mass had the lowest risk of cardiovascular problems and lower total mortality. The authors found that maintaining muscle mass was of the utmost importance "in order to prolong life, even in people who have a high cardiovascular risk."

Respiratory Disease

The *Journal of Clinical Medicine* literature review recounted that 60 percent of patients with respiratory failure who required mechanical ventilation were found to have sarcopenia. In addition, sarcopenia was associated with poorer forced vital capacity (the amount of air that can be forcibly exhaled), which is an accurate measure of lung function.

Cancer

The presence of sarcopenia in cancer patients is ominous. Whether more starting muscle mass means less muscle wasting from the cancer, which is itself a cause of cancer death, or that more starting muscle strength signifies a healthier patient more able to combat their disease, it's clear that having more muscle protects against the complications of cancer. As Bruce Y. Lee put it in a 2018 *Forbes* magazine article, "Maybe one can muscle out cancer." Here are some of the findings in regard to cancer patients with sarcopenia:

> Irrespective of the type of cancer, sarcopenic people with cancer are more likely to experience severe chemotherapy toxicity events.

> For patients with breast cancer, sarcopenia is associated with a shorter time to tumor progression, and those with low muscle mass are significantly less likely to survive from stage 2 or 3 cancer. Additionally, those sarcopenic breast cancer patients who also had a high amount of body fat were 89 percent more likely to have died.

> Sarcopenia is associated with a higher mortality for those with pancreatic cancer.

> Renal cell cancer patients who also have sarcopenia have longer hospital stays, more metastatic sites, and a worsened overall survival rate than those without sarcopenia.

> Sarcopenia is associated with a shorter overall survival for those with bladder (urothelial) cancer.

> Sarcopenic patients receiving radiotherapy for head and neck cancer have a decreased five-year survival rate (67 percent versus 10 percent).

Kidney and Liver Diseases

Patients suffering from kidney disease have much poorer outcomes if they have sarcopenia, while those with end-stage renal disease have an increased risk of death. If someone has both sarcopenia and cirrhosis of the liver, one is more likely to develop hepatic encephalopathy (a build-up of toxicities in the brain).

Hospitalized Patients and Surgical Complications

Even a hospital visit can be more dangerous for those with sarcopenia. Studies show that the presence of sarcopenia in hospitalized elderly patients increases infections acquired during their stay. In fact, hospitalized patients with sarcopenia have an increased risk of death from *all* causes.

And if you are hospitalized for surgery, the disadvantages continue. Following general elective surgery, patients with sarcopenia are more likely to have to go to a rehabilitation or skilled nursing facility. A study examining 170 elderly patients after emergency surgery found sarcopenic patients to have more than three times as many post-operative complications (45 percent versus 15 percent) and to be almost six times more likely to die while in the hospital (23 percent versus 4 percent).

Sarcopenic patients undergoing colorectal procedures have significantly higher 30-day in-hospital mortality rate, and a worse recurrence-free survival rate following stages 1–4 resectable colon surgery. The recurrence-free survival rate is also significantly impacted for endometrial cancer surgery patients with sarcopenia. Patients with sarcopenia that have liver transplant surgery show an increased mortality rate at one and five years post-operatively, and more complications after one year.

Thermoregulation

The loss of muscle mass has serious metabolic consequences due to skeletal muscle's varied and important role in the body. One area of interest is how thermoregulation, the body's maintenance of its internal temperature, may be affected by sarcopenia. In a 2015 article by Jie Yu in the *International Journal of Nursing Sciences*, it was found that changes in thermoregulation, a central component of homeostasis, at the very least may affect energy level and sleep quality.

∗∗∗

As you can see, the mental, medical, surgical, and musculoskeletal problems associated with sarcopenia are vast and wide-ranging. Whether community-based or hospital-based, healthy or sick, the effects can lead to illness, disability, institutionalization, and death. According to one estimate, just a 10 percent reduction in sarcopenia could result in the potential annual savings of $1.1 billion in the United States.

CHAPTER 2

Treating Sarcopenia: Progressive Resistance Exercises

"…exercise therapy is safe and highly effective for sarcopenia."

—Tetsuro Hida and Atsushi Harada, et al., in *Aging and Disease*

While science continues to discover more about the causes and effects of sarcopenia, current research clearly backs up what's long been known—that exercise, especially progressive resistance exercise (PRE), is the cornerstone of any treatment program to battle the ravages of aging.

The essential element of PRE is to continually challenge the muscles to get stronger. You do this by adding to the amount of weight you lift or increasing the resistance of exercise tubing, and by doing more sets as you get stronger.

Remember, at a certain point the strength of the muscles does not appear to be appreciably improved by one's general physical activity level. Of course, if you're real couch potato, then engaging in moderate vigorous physical activity will initially have a positive impact on your muscles. Before long, however, your progress will stall. It seems to be a truth in health and fitness that meaningful gains in strength—whether from muscle, bone, or the cardiovascular system—are only achieved by challenging the body, even if only briefly, to the point of exhaustion. And the evidence certainly indicates that the age-related loss of muscle mass, strength, and power can be counteracted by resistance exercise.

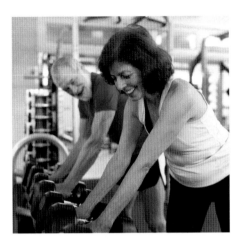

As one 2012 article puts it, "the only strategy that has been shown to be safe and effective [against sarcopenia] is some form of resistance (strength or power) exercise training; this is true even in very old individuals."

Research has also discovered the benefits of a nutritional approach to treating sarcopenia—with proper protein consumption at the forefront—especially when combined with PRE. This and other nutritional, supplemental, and pharmacologic strategies that are showing promise will be discussed in Chapter 6.

Keep in mind that while recent studies proving the beneficial effects of PRE use muscle mass and strength changes for their outcomes, the benefits derived go beyond the musculoskeletal system to affect many other disorders associated with sarcopenia. We'll start with the common and serious condition of osteoporosis.

Osteoporosis and PRE

In a study published in the *Journal of the American Medical Association* examining the effects of high-intensity strength training on osteoporotic fracture risk factors, 39 post-menopausal sedentary women, aged 50 to 70 years, were enrolled. The women were divided into two groups; one group trained two days per week with five different high-intensity strength-training exercises, while the others did not exercise, over the course of a year. The results showed that the women who did strength training:

> showed an increase in femoral neck and lumbar spine bone mineral density.

> preserved total body bone mineral content.

> increased muscle mass.

> increased muscle strength.

> increased dynamic balance.

In contrast, those women who did not exercise:

> had a decrease in bone mineral density in all areas tested.

> showed reduced muscle mass and strength.

> exhibited a decrease in dynamic balance.

The findings were conclusive—high-intensity exercise significantly improves strength and balance while also maintaining bone density for post-menopausal women. One of the most impressive results of this study is that these gains in bone density, muscle strength, and balance were achieved in previously inactive women with just two days a week of strength training.

Increasing Strength and Power with PRE

Power is strength in action, and is a very important attribute needed to right yourself when you begin to fall. But is it hard to achieve? Not at all. With PRE you can get positive results from beginning a resistance exercise program after just one week!

In a 2004 study published in *The Journals of Gerontology: Series A*, eight young adults and seven older adults participated in six weeks of resistance exercise training. Researchers tested the thigh muscle—especially important for balance and preventing falls—by measuring isometric knee extension contractions. The results showed:

> significant increases of the amount of weight subjects could lift one time (strength) and in the speed at which muscles could generate force (power) in one week.

> that the older adults increased their strength by 36 percent, compared to 29 percent by the younger ones.

> that the older adults increased their power by 49 percent, compared to 15 percent by the younger ones, after the six-week program.

The results illustrate not only that strength *and* power improved, but how quickly you can achieve fitness gains. The more science discovers about the body, the more we learn how fast the body reacts when physically challenged. This was also illustrated in my book, *Staying Young with Interval Training*, regarding the impressive early gains in health and fitness that occur after beginning a high-intensity aerobic exercise program.

In the same vein, this study also reveals the impressive gains the older participants enjoyed when compared to the younger ones, a phenomenon that is also seen in the interval training studies. While this likely reflects the fact that older individuals have more to gain than their younger counterparts, nonetheless it illustrates the impressive health benefits that older individuals can achieve.

The Elderly and PRE

Are you ever too old to start exercising? In a word, no! Take the 1994 study reported in the *New England Journal of Medicine*. With the goal of strengthening the knee and hip extensor muscles, researchers asked 100 frail men and women living in nursing homes, with a mean age of 87 years old, to lift weights three days per week for 10 weeks. The amount of weight used was significant, set at 80 percent of the amount that each participant could manage to lift just one time; the amount was increased each training session as the participants got stronger. Impressively, 94 percent of the participants completed the study, proving that even frail and elderly people can perform challenging exercises. The study found that:

> muscle strength increased by 113 percent.

> walking speed (sometimes called the sixth vital sign because of how predictive it is to health status) and stair-climbing power increased significantly.

> muscle size increased (cross-sectional thigh muscle mass was larger).

> participants increased their level of *spontaneous* physical activity; these previously frail people felt better to the point they ate more food and had more energy for activity.

The researchers concluded that even with very elderly and/or frail people, high-intensity resistance exercises really do improve muscle strength. This translates into an improved ability to perform everyday activities and better quality of life.

Are You Ever Too Sick?

It's not only frail elderly people who can benefit from resistance training. Weak and chronically ill elderly patients can also get stronger, according to a 2018 study in the *European Journal of Physical and Rehabilitation Medicine*. This strengthening study involved 54 women and men, with an average age of 82 years, all living in retirement care facilities, and all with various health impairments. After six months of elastic band resistance training, the study reported significantly enhanced muscle quality of the lower extremities, prompting the authors to conclude: "Elastic band resistance training could be safely used to improve muscle quality even in old people with impaired health status. Weak and chronically ill participants benefited the most from this training."

Is It Ever Too Late?

As we discussed in Chapter 1, a significant percentage of older adults fall and fracture their hip, almost a third of whom will die within a year, with many more suffering long-term disability and functional loss. Since it was also discovered that sarcopenia is present in a large percentage of hip fracture patients, an important question arises: Is it too late to intervene after a hip fracture, to use resistance training as a tool to reduce the disability and death that so frequently follows?

As reported in the *Journal of the American Medical Directors Association*, a 2012 study was performed on 124 outpatients who had surgery for a hip fracture. The participants agreed to 12 months of supervised high-intensity weight lifting along with nutritional, cognitive, and social support. Compared to controls who did not weight lift or engage in the other treatment interventions, the people who did weight lifting reduced their risk of death by 81 percent and admissions to nursing homes by 84 percent. In addition, the weight lifters discovered they were better able to perform everyday tasks with significantly less reliance on assistive devices.

Now those are impressive benefits. Not only did PRE drastically reduce the post-hip-fracture mortality rate, but also it improved quality of life by keeping patients independent and out of nursing homes.

Do the Benefits Last?

A study published in the *Journal of Rehabilitation Medicine* revisited a group of men and women four years after they had participated in a study using PRE training to strengthen their leg muscles. At the time of the initial study, each participant had been post-stroke and trained twice a week for just ten weeks. Impressively, the gains in strength enjoyed by the training group at the time of the initial study remained four years later. This prompted the authors to conclude that PRE is an effective method to improve muscle strength with long-term benefits.

Participants trained just twice a week, for ten weeks—20 exercise sessions in total—and the beneficial effects of PRE on the muscles were still present four years later! As you can see by this and the other studies cited in this chapter, the evidence clearly indicates that the age-related loss of muscle mass, strength, and power can be effectively counteracted by exercise, regardless of age, living conditions, and, to a certain extent, health status. Strategies to combat sarcopenia, including PRE, are therefore essential, not only to maintain and build muscle, but also to improve balance, reduce falls, decrease the risk of depression and dementia, reduce post-operative complications, prevent and reduce chronic disease, and increase the quantity and quality of life.

STAYING IN THE GAME

Many of PRE's health benefits result directly from better fitness—the increased strength and power of the muscles, and the improved stamina of the cardiovascular and respiratory systems. One of the fitness benefits of strength training that is not always appreciated, however, is the ability to continue exercising when others may have to stop. I've met many older patients in my office whose exercise program didn't include weight training, and at some point they had been forced to give up their aerobic exercise because of chronic and debilitating hip, knee, or back pain. A stronger musculoskeletal system is vital to protect the joints and makes these exercise-related injuries less likely.

Weight and PRE

The increased muscle-to-fat ratio from PRE also aids in weight loss. Since muscle burns more calories than fat does, weight training increases the body's metabolism, improving weight management and body reshaping for those interested in looking more fit. And women need not worry about looking too muscular, since their hormonal balance typically won't allow it.

Fitness experts also tout the benefits of the after-burn effect—the ability muscle has to continue burning calories long after a workout has officially ended. Perhaps more so than other forms of exercise, weight training fires up the cellular mechanisms responsible for metabolism for hours after your session officially ends.

In contrast, a real problem for many older people is difficulty gaining weight, and they can become too thin. This is significant because their weight loss can reduce muscle mass and lead to sarcopenia. Fortunately, strength training can reverse this trend and put the needed pounds back on since muscle weighs more than fat. According to *Medicine and Science in Sports and Exercise*, a review of studies demonstrated that older men gained more than 2 pounds in lean body mass on average after PRE training. If you're in this category, the information on protein and nutrition in Chapter 6 should also be very beneficial to your gaining weight.

CHAPTER 3

How to Strengthen Muscles

"I do it as a therapy. I do it as something to keep me alive. We all need a little discipline. Exercise is my discipline."

—Jack LaLanne

While weight training has been shown to cause relatively few injuries as compared to other sports—with no significant differences due to age or sex—muscle strains can occur when you begin any new exercise program. Therefore, if you're new to weight training, it's important to get into the nuts and bolts of how to build muscle to minimize the risk of injury and maximize the benefits.

Safety First

First and foremost, getting medically cleared for weight-training exercise is a good idea for all adults, and it's especially important if you're pregnant, have a medical condition, take medication, or have balance issues. Use any health information you gather from your medical visit for comparison later, to see how your health has improved after you've been exercising for a while.

Although weight training has proven to be safe, the screening questions that follow can be used to further identify if you're at high risk for an adverse event. This test is just a guide to help make your experience more positive; it offers no guarantee, and shouldn't replace professional medical advice:

1. Do you have a heart condition or have you suffered a stroke?

2. Do you have unexplained chest pain or pressure during activity or at rest?

3. Do you ever feel faint or have dizzy spells during exercise, resulting in a loss of balance?

4. Have you had an asthma attack that required urgent medical assistance in the last 12 months?

5. If diabetic, have you had difficulty controlling your blood sugar levels in the last three months?

6. Do you have a muscle, bone, or joint problem that your doctor told you may worsen by engaging in physical activity?

7. Do you have a recent injury or healing wound?

8. Do you have any other medical problems or take medications that may make exercising dangerous for you?

If you answered YES to any of the eight questions above, seek assistance and medical clearance from a healthcare professional. If you answered NO to all eight questions, and have no other concerns, you can start a light-intensity exercise program.

EXERCISE AND PAIN: WHEN TO SEEK HELP

- Stop exercising immediately and seek medical help if you experience chest pain or pressure, difficulty breathing, or become dizzy or light-headed, weak, nauseous, or have other abnormal or unsteady feelings.
- While soreness after exercising for a day or two is normal, especially when engaging in new routines, stop and consult your physician if pain is sharp or if discomfort lasts longer than a day.
- Joint pain, swelling, redness, or skin that's warm to touch can be the result of inflammation and requires rest, ice, and medical help if prolonged.

Proper Form

Proper form is the most important element to building muscle. Muscles are arranged and work in very specific directions and manners. Moving in a way that compromises this—usually the result of poor posture or poor technique—creates tension and strain on the muscles and joints. Now stress those strained areas with weights and resistance and you can develop tendinitis, bursitis, and soft-tissue sprains.

Breathing properly is an important aspect of good form. Don't hold your breath for any length of time. Gently exhale during times of exertion and inhale during rest.

While we'll talk more about proper form when describing the specific exercises, it's never a bad idea—especially if you're just starting out in weight training—to get the advice of a fitness expert. Whether for an initial consult or on an ongoing basis, a trainer can help you master the basics of form to make your experience more enjoyable.

If you'd rather go it alone, however, feel free. Studies have demonstrated that home-based exercises are often as effective as those supervised by an expert. A 2017 study cited in the journal *Clinical Rehabilitation* compared supervised PRE training and unsupervised home-based PRE following knee replacement surgery, and found equally impressive improvements in power and function in both groups.

One of the fun parts of beginning any exercise routine is the big gains in strength you'll see in the first days and weeks. And while this will encourage you to continue, avoid the temptation to increase the workload too soon. Going slowly in the beginning is essential to ingraining proper form and avoiding injury. Temper your enthusiasm and move up only when you can easily handle your current level.

Warming Up and Dynamic Stretches

Warming up before exercising is always a good idea. And when the exercise involves weights and resistance training, it's a must. While this is true for all ages, it's even more important for middle-aged and older adults to minimize the risk of injury. Warming up gets the blood flowing, the heart pumping, the muscles and other soft tissues warm and more pliable, increases the range of motion of joints, and gets you mentally prepared for the workout to come.

You only need a 10- to 15-minute warm-up and there are several ways to accomplish this. I recommend starting with 5 minutes of light aerobic exercise—walking, cycling, skipping rope, or just moving in place—followed by 8 to 10 dynamic stretches. Finish off with a few of the strengthening exercises you'll be doing using light weights or just your body weight. If you want, you can also mix in some static stretches (see page 43). This routine will prepare the muscles for work and may even improve your performance to get the most out of your workouts.

Keep a relaxed posture when doing dynamic stretches. Begin doing the movements slowly and deliberately. Do about 10 repetitions of each movement (on each side, if applicable), in each direction, one time through. Unlike static stretches, dynamic stretch positions aren't held in place, just performed in a fluid, smooth range of motion. Hold onto the back of a chair or counter for stability, if necessary.

Arms and Shoulders

Arm Circles

1–2. Sit or stand with good posture. Bring both arms straight up and, in a continuous motion, bring them backward, down, then forward, forming a circle.

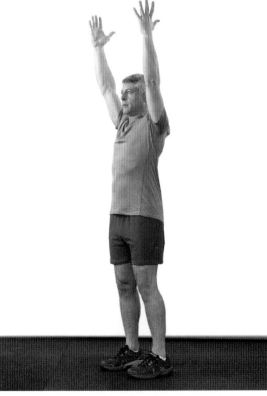
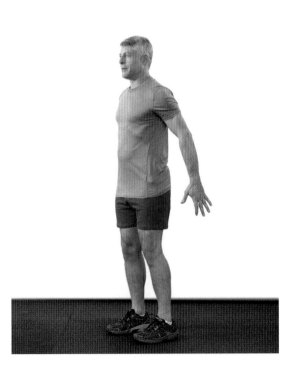

Repeat in the other direction.

Wrist Circles

1. Sit or stand with good posture. Clasp your hands together in front of your chest with fingers interlaced, palms touching, and thumbs on top. Keep your shoulders relaxed and elbows bent at about 90 degrees.

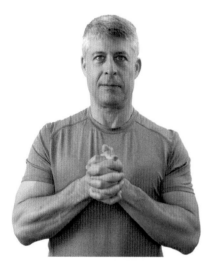

2–3. Rotate your clasped hands in a full circle, then immediately retrace the circle in the reverse direction to return to starting position.

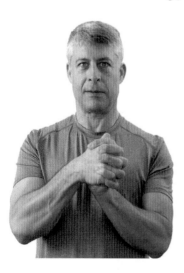

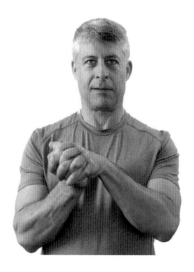

Shoulder Blade Mobility

1. Start on all fours with your hands beneath your shoulders. Bring your left hand up and lightly place it on the back of your head with your elbow pointing to the side.

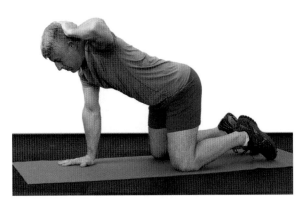

2. Now bring your left elbow down so that it points toward the floor, rotating your head and shoulder with it.

3. After a brief pause, move your elbow back up as far as you can comfortably go, rotating your head and shoulder with it, until your elbow is parallel to or above the floor, if possible.

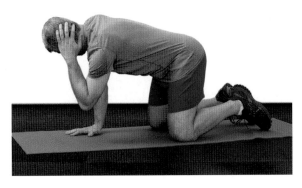

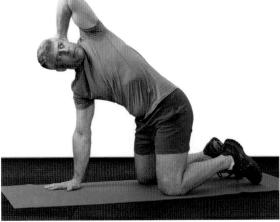

Switch sides and repeat.

Upper and Lower Back

Trunk Side Bend

1. Stand with your feet shoulder-width apart. Raise your left arm straight over your head and place your right hand on your hip. Bend your trunk laterally to the right as far as it will comfortably go.

2. Return to the center, switch arm positions, and then bend laterally to the left.

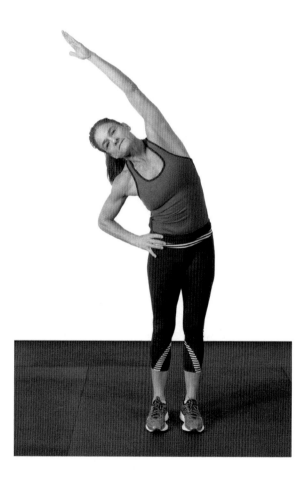

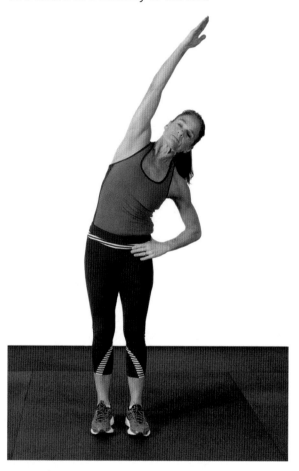

Return to starting position.

Trunk Rotation

1. Stand with your feet shoulder-width apart, arms out to the sides and parallel to the ground, elbows fully bent, and fists touching your chest. Rotate your upper body and head to the right as far as you can comfortably go so that you're looking over your right shoulder.

2. In a smooth motion, move back to the center and continue rotating to the left.

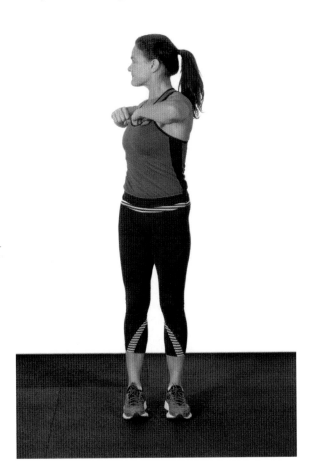

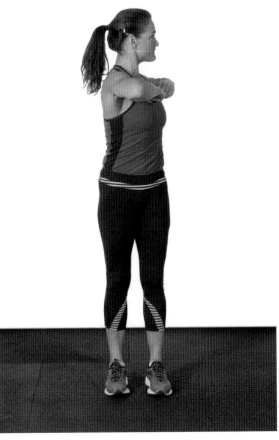

Return to starting position.

Core

Glute Bridge

1. Lie on your back on the floor with knees bent, feet flat on the ground, and arms by your sides.

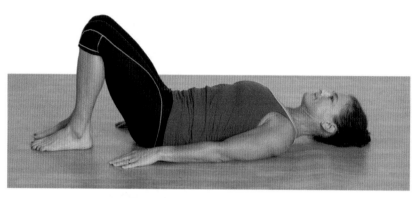

2. Press your weight into your heels and lift your pelvis up off the floor, creating a straight line from your trunk to your knees. Keep your head and neck relaxed as you tighten your glutes.

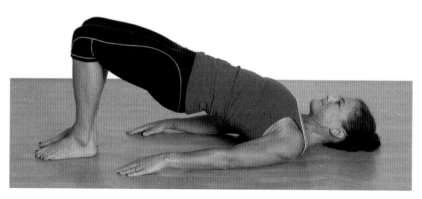

Hold briefly, then slowly lower your pelvis back down to starting position.

Inchworm

1. Start in a downward dog yoga pose, with your legs and arms straight and your hips high up in the air.

2. Keeping your legs and arms straight, walk your hands forward until your arms are under your shoulders and your body forms a straight line from head to toe (top position of a push-up).

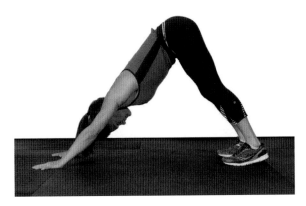

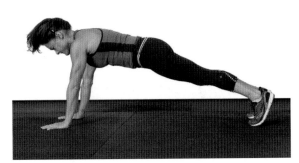

3. After a brief pause, walk your feet forward until they reach your hands, then slowly raise your body until you're standing tall.

4. Bending at the hips, not your lower back, reach your hands to the floor. Bend your knees if necessary.

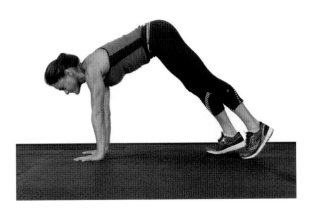

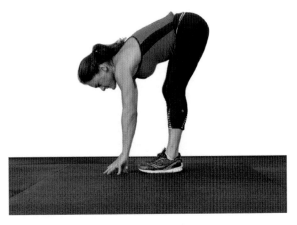

Walk your hands forward until you return to downward dog and repeat.

Lower Body

Hip Swings

1. Stand with your legs hip-width apart and hold onto a counter, wall, or other stable object for support. Keeping your left leg straight, slowly swing it forward to a comfortable height.

2. Keeping your upper body straight and abdominals slightly tightened, allow your leg to slowly come back down before swinging it behind you.

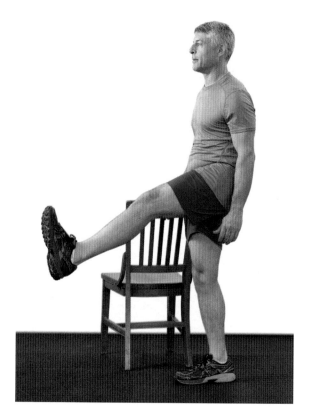 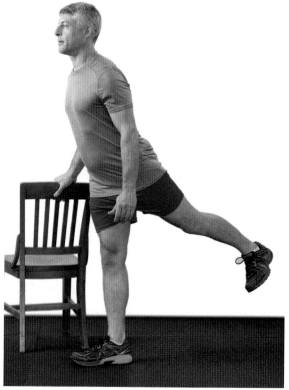

Repeat and then switch sides.

Knee to Chest

1. Stand with good posture and bring your right knee up toward your chest, grabbing your shin if you can as it comes close.

2. After a brief pause, let the right leg go and bring the left knee up.

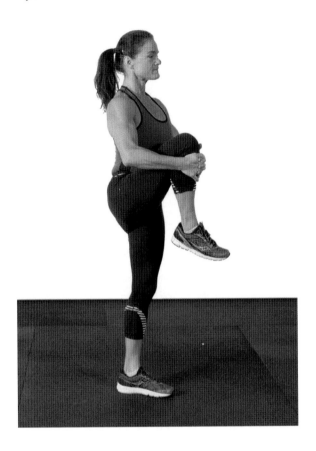

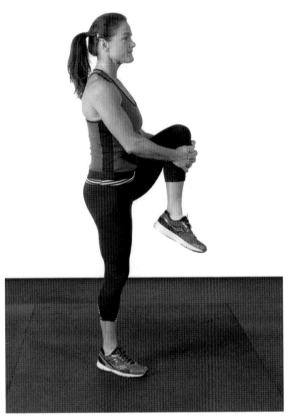

Knee Circles

1. From a standing position, your feet a couple of inches apart, bend slightly at the hips and knees and place your hands on your thighs just above your knees. (Remember, whenever you bend at the hips, you should be aware of your butt sticking out behind you and your lower back being straight.)

2. Slowly begin to make small- to medium-sized circles with your knees, first clockwise, and then counterclockwise. (Don't worry if you hear some minor pops and clicks coming from your joints as you do the exercise.)

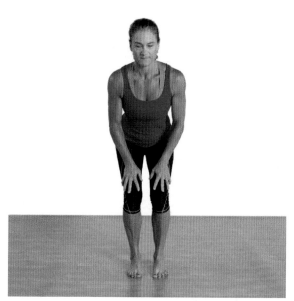

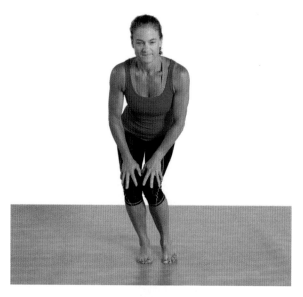

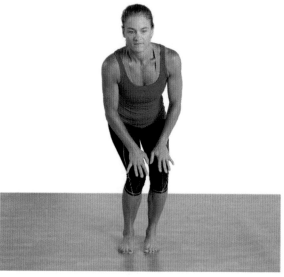

Do 10 to 15 circles in each direction.

Cooling Down and Static Stretches

The goal of cooling down after a workout is to allow your cardiovascular system to return gradually to its pre-exercise level. While cooling down has not been proven to be mandatory, it has been the experience of many exercisers—myself included—that abruptly ending an intense workout can leave one feeling lightheaded, dizzy, or nauseous. Blood vessels dilate during a workout, which concentrates blood in the muscles. Stopping all activity before the blood has had a chance to redistribute throughout the body may make blood less available for the brain and other organs, creating those ill feelings.

A 5- to 10-minute cool-down is usually all you need to slow down the vascular system, heart rate, and breathing rate. Cooling down doesn't actually reduce post-workout muscle soreness, but it is a good time to do some flexibility exercises. Limber up the body with some light aerobic exercise or foam-rolling (there are plenty of resources for foam-rolling, including in my book *Staying Young with Interval Training*), and choose some of the following static stretches to increase flexibility and joint range of motion.

Studies prove that you only have to do a static stretch once per session to benefit, but you do need to hold it for a minimum of 30 seconds.

Neck Stretch

The Position: Lie on your back on the floor and let your head relax for a few seconds. Reach back and place the fingers of both hands in the space behind your neck, with your fingertips touching or fingers interlocked, and very gently move them up along the floor until they contact the back of your resting head. Keep moving your fingers up, pushing—or sliding—the back of your head up, feeling the back of the neck elongating. You may also notice that this movement tilts your head down and tucks your chin slightly.

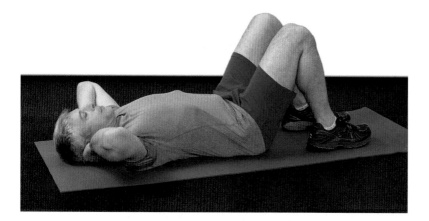

Shoulder Stretch

The Position: Lie on the floor face up and extend your arms straight out to the sides.

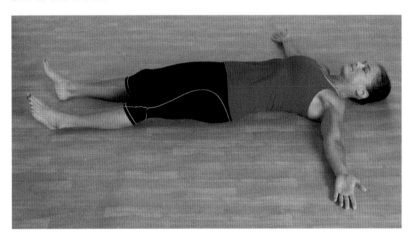

NOTE: If you don't feel a stretch in the shoulder or chest muscles when lying on the floor, try lying with the roller along the length of your spine. A rolled-up towel or foam roller will do nicely. Your head should be supported by the roller itself or with a pillow of equal height. As long as you keep them on the floor, you can vary the position of your arms (lower toward your hips, higher toward your head) to stretch different parts of the chest and shoulder muscles.

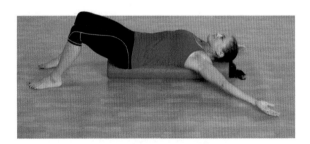

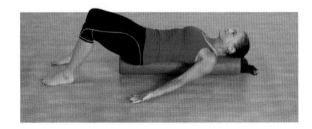

Lower-Back Stretch

1. Lie flat on your stomach with your forehead resting on the backs of your crossed hands. Relax your belly and feel the natural curve of your lower back. This may provide a sufficient stretch on its own.

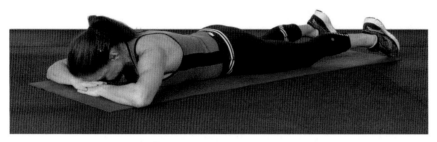

2. Come up onto your elbows (the sphinx pose in yoga) or the palms of your hands (the cobra yoga pose). Remember, it's more important to relax the belly and let the lower back stretch gently than it is to try to go up higher.

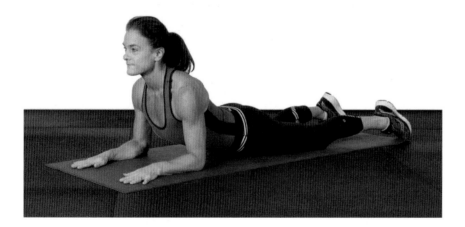

Hip Stretch

1. Sit in a chair and rest your left ankle on top of your right thigh, just above the knee.

2. Gently hinge at the waist, leaning your upper body forward until you feel a stretch in your thigh/butt area. Make sure to keep your upper and lower back straight rather than letting them round. In other words, don't slump!

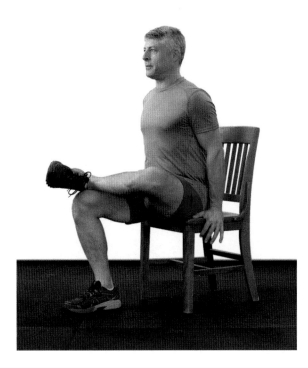

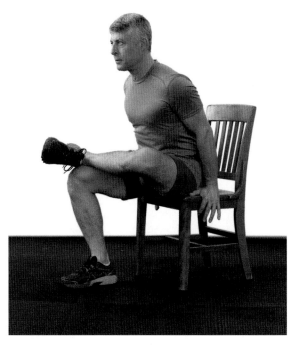

Switch sides and repeat.

47

Front of the Thigh Stretch

The Position: Stand with your left hand holding the back of a chair or other stable object for balance. Bend your right knee and grab your right ankle behind you with your right hand. Your right knee should be pointing down toward the floor. While holding the ankle in place, stand nice and tall, pushing your pelvis slightly forward. You should feel a gentle stretch in the front of your right thigh.

Switch sides and repeat.

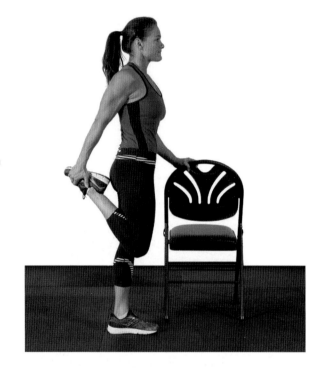

Back of the Thigh Stretch

The Position: Stand with your right leg straight out in front of you with the heel resting on a chair seat, ottoman, or similar object, and bend forward at the hip joint. Don't slouch or round your back. You should feel a gentle stretch in the back of your right thigh.

Switch sides and repeat.

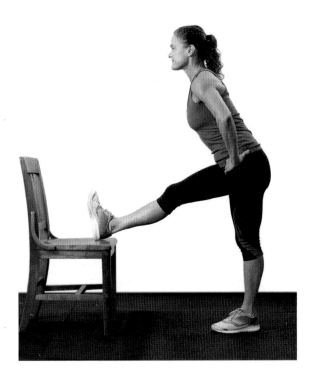

Calf Stretch

The Position: Stand a few feet away from a chair, wall, or other stable object. Step forward with your right leg, bending at the knee as you lean your body forward and hinge at the left ankle joint. Reach for the stable object with your outstretched arms. Make sure to keep your back straight as you lean forward and keep your left heel firmly planted on the ground. Move closer to or farther from the object until you feel a good stretch in the left calf muscle.

Switch sides and repeat.

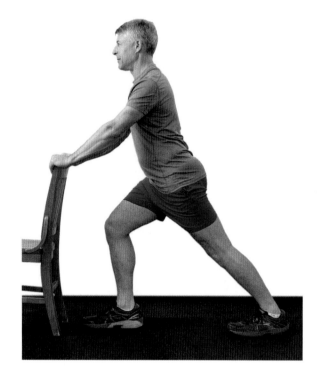

Shin Stretch

1. Stand and hold onto a wall, chair, or counter for stability. Bend both knees slightly and place your left foot a few inches behind your right, with your left heel in the air and toes touching the ground (like a ballet dancer).

2. Pull your left leg forward without your left toes moving from their spot, causing your left heel to move forward, until a stretch is felt in the right shin.

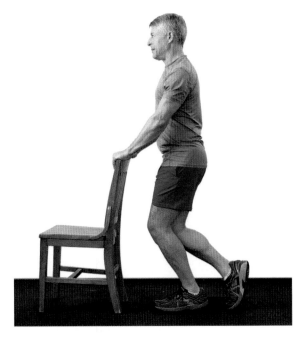

Switch sides and repeat.

Note: If you're flexible, this stretch can also be done while sitting on the floor, bending your legs underneath you, toes pointing behind you, with your butt sitting back on your heels. This stretches both shins at once.

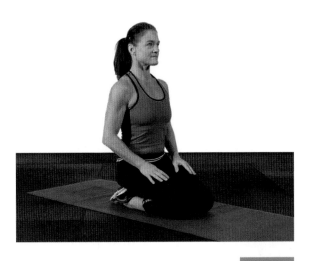

CHAPTER 4

The Program

"Those who do not find time for exercise will have to find time for illness."

—Edward Stanley

Now is the time to grow stronger, not older. There is no reason that this can't be your best year yet—the year you get fitter and healthier. You can gain muscle, lose weight, reshape your body, gain more energy, increase your stamina and confidence, and at the same time lower your blood pressure and improve your cholesterol and triglyceride profiles. And most importantly, reverse any current muscle loss and decrease the likelihood you'll develop sarcopenia, with its myriad physical, mental, medical, and surgical complications.

"The program" is your overall fitness plan and the workouts within it. A PRE program utilizing the latest research to optimally train the musculoskeletal system is included. Of course, one size does not fit all, and options are included to tailor the program to your needs based on your fitness level, health status, and goals.

The most important part of any program is showing up. All efforts will be rewarded, and it has been my experience that having small goals is a great way of getting started. I like to trick myself by putting on my sneakers and agreeing to just do some warm-ups, and then maybe a couple of exercises. Once I've begun, I frequently find I get more in the mood and go on to do a full workout.

The American College of Sports Medicine (ACSM), one of the leading sports medicine and exercise science organizations, recommends a total fitness program that includes regular aerobic exercise, progressive resistance training (the cornerstone of the sarcopenia reversal and prevention program), stretching exercises for flexibility and joint range of motion, and exercises for balance, agility, and coordination (yoga and tai chi are examples of these types of exercise).

Implementing this program will not only transform your life, but also, according to the Centers for Disease Control and Prevention, will make you one of only 23 percent of U.S. adults spending the recommended amount of time doing cardiovascular and strength-training exercises.

Here is a two-week sample exercise program based on the ACSM's recommendations. Since my goal is to get the most effective workout in the shortest amount of time, however, I've significantly decreased the time that they recommend for exercising. Studies demonstrate that one set of progressive resistance training and 10 minutes of aerobic (HIIT) workouts per session are very effective. If you want to add a second set, or another high-intensity interval to your training, just be prepared to spend a little extra time.

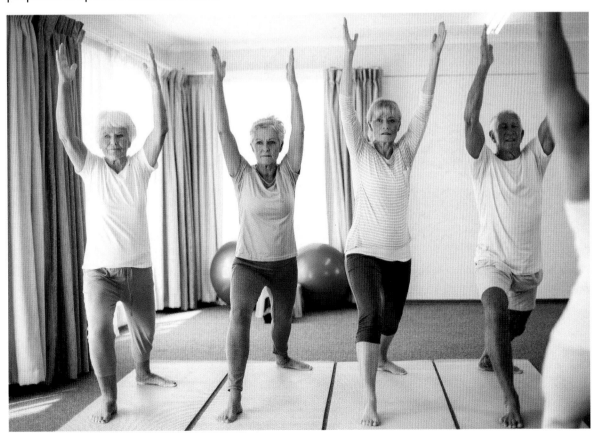

Week 1

Monday: Warm-up, 15 minutes PRE, cool-down

Tuesday: Rest, stretching, or moderate-paced exercise

Wednesday: Warm-up, 10 minutes HIIT, cool-down

Thursday: Balance exercises, yoga, tai chi

Friday: Warm-up, 15 minutes PRE, cool-down

Saturday: Rest, stretching, or moderate-paced exercise

Sunday: Warm-up, 10 minutes HIIT, cool-down

Week 2

Monday: Rest, stretching, or moderate-paced exercise

Tuesday: Warm-up, 15 minutes PRE, cool-down

Wednesday: Balance exercises, yoga, tai chi

Thursday: Warm-up, 10 minutes HIIT, cool-down

Friday: Warm-up, 15 minutes PRE, cool-down

Saturday: Rest, stretching, or moderate-paced exercise

Sunday: Warm-up, 10 minutes HIIT, cool-down

You can also add a day or two of longer moderate-paced exercises—walking, biking, swimming—on one of your rest days. While static stretching should be part of the warm-up and/or cool down for PRE and HIIT exercise, I recommend you also do some stretching on your rest days. See my book *End Everyday Pain for 50+* for a quick 10-minute-a-day flexibility program.

Exercises

The exercises are the activities, or movements, engaged in to improve the body. For our purposes—to strengthen the body and prevent or reverse sarcopenia—the general recommendation is to perform six to nine total exercises, working the major muscle groups of the whole body, against the resistance of free weights, elastic bands, or your body weight. The focus should be on the large muscles of the legs, hips, back, chest, shoulders, and arms. Chapter 5 lists the exercises, divided into upper body, core, and lower body. Pick and choose two or three from each category, changing them periodically. Try to strengthen the front and back of the body in a balanced way. For example, if you choose exercises that strengthen the front of the thighs—the quadriceps muscles using leg extensions—also strengthen the back of the thighs—the hamstring muscles using leg curls.

Exercises are sometimes classified as either compound or isolation exercises. Most of the exercises included in this book are compound exercises.

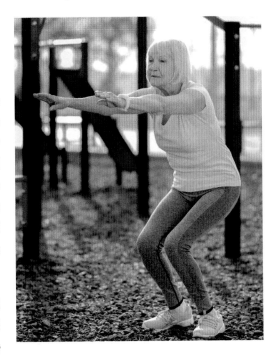

Compound exercises target the major muscle groups and utilize multiple muscles and joints during the exercise. Squats are a good example of this as they exercise many major muscles of the legs, hips, and butt, as well as the ankle, knee, and hip joints. Because they work such a large area, compound exercises are efficient and safer. They are also more practical and functional, in that they more closely mimic activities we do in everyday life.

Isolation exercises target a specific muscle or two, and usually involve a single joint—biceps curls are a good example of this. While they are useful, they are not the major part of this resistance training since the isolating nature of these exercises makes them riskier, and less applicable to daily activities. They should typically be done at the end of a workout, after the muscles have been thoroughly warmed up from compound exercises.

Intensity

The intensity of a workout is a combination of the amount of weight lifted, or resistance, and the targeted number of repetitions. If you're just beginning a PRE program, or getting back into one after a long layoff, start with lower intensity by choosing a weight, or resistance setting, that allows you to do more repetitions comfortably. While this is designed to prevent injury, the higher number of repetitions will still tone and strengthen your body. As you gain experience, you can ratchet it up to a moderate intensity by adding more weight and decreasing the number of repetitions.

Repetitions

Repetitions, or reps for short, are the number of times you lift the weight, or pull the tube, within a single session, without taking more than a brief rest in between. Start out at 15 to 18 reps, working at an effort level of 5 to 6 out of 10. Gradually increase the intensity until you can only do 12 to 15 reps at a time.

At some point—usually in a month or two—you'll find that with stronger muscles the exercises get easier. Once you're doing two to four more reps than the targeted range, it's time to increase the resistance to bring you back down. If you're using free weights, adding about 5 percent to the weight will usually do the job. Ultimately, the goal for a moderately intense workout is to be doing 8 to 12 reps. Remember, the range you choose means that you fatigue within that number, where doing one more rep wouldn't be possible while maintaining good form.

Velocity

The speed at which you perform an exercise should be deliberate and controlled. The range of time to complete one repetition of an exercise is about 6 to 9 seconds, with a 1- to 2-second rest between reps.

Sets

A group of repetitions forms a set. While only a brief rest occurs between reps, there is always a longer rest period between sets—assuming you're doing more than one during a workout session. One set of each exercise is all you should be doing in the beginning. You will get stronger and make progress while minimizing the risk of overworking your muscles. Most fitness experts agree, however, that after an initial beginner phase, moving up to two to three sets is necessary to gain maximal strength.

That said, a recent study published in *Medicine and Science in Sports and Exercise* recruited 34 men to test the impact of differing numbers of resistance training sets on the muscles. The men were divided into three groups. All did the same seven exercises, for 8 to 12 repetitions until exhaustion, three times a week. The difference was the number of sets each group did: one, three, or five. After the eight-week program, all three groups enjoyed significant increases in strength and endurance—with no difference between them! That's right, gains in strength and endurance did not change based on the number of sets performed, only the size of the muscles, which did get bigger when more sets were performed. Considering that one, three, and five sets took 13, 40, and 70 minutes, respectively, it's hard to argue with doing just one set. As the authors put it, "Marked increase in strength and endurance can be attained by resistance-trained individuals with just three 13-minute weekly sessions over an eight-week period, and these gains are similar to that achieved with a substantially greater time commitment."

Rest

The most important rest interval with PRE is the day between workout sessions. Always take a rest day between training sessions to allow the muscles to recover. The other important rest period is the one between exercise sets, if you're doing more than one set. The research points to a 3- to 5-minute rest between sets to meet the twin goals of gaining strength and safety.

Frequency

Recent research on exercise and health points to a higher-intensity, less frequent workout approach. Just like with cardiovascular training—and described in my book *Staying Young with Interval Training*—significant benefits from PRE training can be had in less time than previously thought. One PRE session per week will likely translate into significant gains in muscle strength and effectively combat sarcopenia. That said, while the added time commitment may not translate equally into added benefits, doing an additional training session or two per week will boost muscle strength and mass. Just be sure to always take a rest day in between multiple training sessions per week.

Varying Your Routine

People engaged in strength training sometimes experience a slowdown in their progress—likely due to the body's amazing ability to adapt to stress—typically within the first five months of a strength-training program. To prevent this, you can alter your workout routine in several ways:

> Vary the exercises: In the following chapter, you'll find many exercise options to strengthen the muscles within the regions of the body. Periodically change the exercises to challenge the muscles in slightly different ways. Mix it up.

> Vary the intensity: Every couple of weeks or so, vary the intensity of your workouts by straying outside the recommended range of 8 to 12 reps, adjusting the weight accordingly. In other words, occasionally do fewer repetitions—maybe 6 to 8—with heavier weight or more resistance, and at other times go for more repetitions—maybe 15 to 18—with lighter weight

or less resistance. You can also vary the intensity by changing the number of sets performed, perhaps just one with the heavier weights, and three with the lighter.

> Vary the body regions worked: This is also known as a split workout. After you've gained some experience and conditioned your body by doing whole-body workouts, consider dedicating training days to specific areas, like the lower body. By splitting up your workout in this way, you can do all 8 to 10 exercises on one region. And as the other regions are resting that day, you can train more days during the week.

As some of these changes involve more intensity, you might consider enlisting the help of an exercise trainer.

Tools and Equipment

Whether at home or at the gym, pick the tools and equipment that are convenient for your lifestyle and that you enjoy using. And by removing as many obstacles as you can identify—the travel time to the gym or the isolation of a home workout—you'll keep exercising when perhaps you'd rather not. Some of the more common training-tool options are:

Body weights: The cheapest, most convenient, and safest method to weight train. Ideal for beginners and as warm-ups for all levels. It has been around since the beginning of time.

Free weights: Dumbbells, ankle weights, barbells, kettlebells, and others. Free weights have been around a long time and are the mainstays of most programs due to their ease of use and versatility.

Resistance or exercise tubing, or bands: Popular because you can creatively use them to strengthen the entire body, and they are inexpensive and portable. They come in many shapes, sizes, and resistance levels. I use a version of clip-tube resistance bands that have clips, or carabiners, to easily attach the resistance tubes to handles and ankle straps, as well as to a handy door anchor.

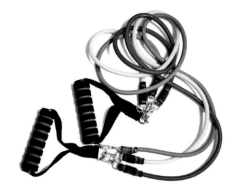

Medicine balls and sandbags: These weighted objects can be used to develop strength and power, using them through broad ranges of motion.

Exercise tubing with carabiners.

Weight machines and gym equipment: Great for beginners because they are relatively safe even when used alone, and have adjustable seats and other features to aid proper form.

Log book: Recording the specifics of your exercise routine—including the amount of weight used, and the number of repetitions and sets—will help you remember your current level as well as to chart your progress. In addition to the details of your workout, scheduling your training sessions will help you remember to do them. I also recommend that you write down your *whys*—the reasons you're exercising—for motivation to keep you devoting your time and energy when obstacles appear.

Optional gear: There are a number of other items that can make your workout more comfortable and enjoyable such as:

> Lightweight supportive sneakers

> Floor mat

> Water bottle

> Push-up handles to avoid wrist strain

> Knee braces to support arthritic knees until they're stronger

> Foam roller for cool-down exercises

CHAPTER 5

The Exercises

"…what a disgrace it is for a man to grow old without ever seeing the beauty and strength of which his body is capable."
—Socrates

If you're new to resistance training, review Chapter 4 for information about the number of repetitions and sets to do, as well as about using less intensity as you're developing strength and experience. While you want to be feeling the work by those last few reps, don't worry if you're not fatigued by the last one. Eventually, that's the goal of PRE, but for now you want to slowly get your muscles in shape and focus on good form.

Never begin resistance training with cold muscles. Do the dynamic stretches starting on page 32 before you begin. Warming up and cooling down are both important activities to maximize the benefits—and minimize the injuries—from resistance training.

Here are some other tips and reminders:

1. Choose 2 to 3 exercises from each body region—upper body, core, and lower body—for a total of 6 to 9. The whole-body workout approach is recommended unless you have a knee, hip, or shoulder problem that currently needs rest; in that case, work around the issue.

2. If you're looking to exercise but time is short, prioritize the lower body since leg strength plays the additional role of keeping balance, avoiding falls, and maintaining independent living as you age.

3. Always give your muscles at least a day off to recover between workouts, allowing them to rest, repair, and grow.

4. And don't forget your log book.

You'll *love* the results!

The exercises in this chapter include those with dumbbells, medicine balls, and resistance bands/tubes. Resistance tubes or bands are great for beginners to tone and build strength. At a certain point, however, switching to superbands—heavy-duty resistance bands—or dumbbells may be needed for PRE to continue to build strength.

When the exercises are for the legs or arms, one side is described. Do the requisite number of repetitions in a row, then switch, and do the other leg or arm.

Neither the number of repetitions, nor the amount of weight or resistance to use, is specified in the exercises described here, since it varies based on your current fitness level.

SHOULDER STRENGTHENING

The backhand/forehand tennis exercises and Thumbs Up exercises (pages 64–69) are important to strengthen the shoulders and avoid many of the problems that older adults get in their shoulders, a result of the rounding that occurs over time. They *must* be done slowly and carefully, with good shoulders-back posture and with minimal weight to avoid straining the muscles. STOP if any pain occurs during the exercises.

Upper Body

These upper-body exercises work many muscles at once in the upper body, including the deltoid and rotator cuff muscles of the shoulders, the pectoralis muscles of the chest, the rhomboid muscles of the upper back, and the trapezius muscle that covers the whole region.

Overhead Press with Weights

This exercise can also be done while sitting.

1. Stand with good posture, feet shoulder-width apart. With an overhand grip, hold a dumbbell in your right hand at shoulder level, palm facing forward and elbow pointing to the floor. Keep your left arm relaxed at your side.

2. Exhale and extend your right arm in a straight line toward the ceiling, keeping your elbow slightly tucked so it doesn't flare out to the side. Stop short of locking the elbow at the top. Don't overarch your lower back.

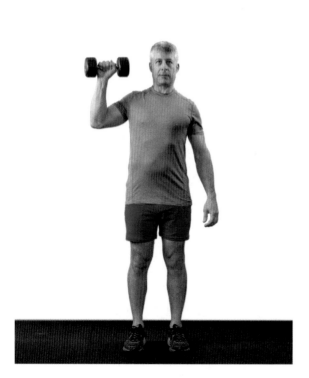

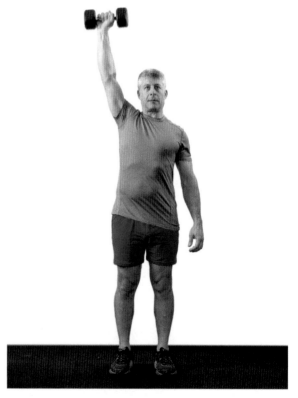

Inhale and slowly return to starting position.

Switch sides and repeat.

Overhead Press with Resistance Tube

1. Stand with good posture, and step one foot forward about two feet into a staggered, stable stance. Place the center of the resistance tube under your front foot. (You can also anchor it low on a door or other immovable, sturdy object behind you.) Grab a handle with each hand, palms facing forward, and raise them to shoulder height, elbows tucked close to your sides and forearms pointing toward the ceiling. Engage your core by tightening your abdominal muscles, keeping your back straight and chest up and slightly forward.

2. Exhale and press both hands straight up over your head, stopping just short of locking your elbows.

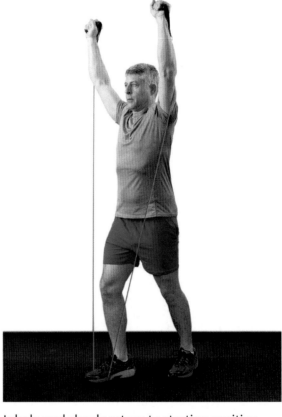

Inhale and slowly return to starting position.

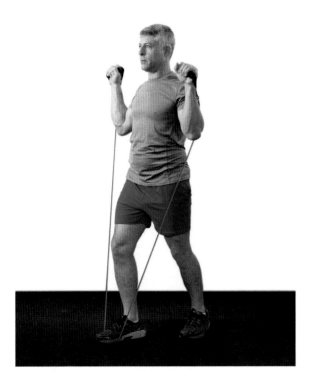

Tennis Backhand with Weights

Do this exercise slowly and carefully, with good shoulders-back posture and with minimal weight to avoid straining the muscles. STOP if any pain occurs.

1. Lie on your right side with your right arm on the floor extended straight up over your head and place a small pillow or rolled-up towel under your right armpit. Hold a weight in your left hand with your left forearm tight across your stomach and elbow bent to 90 degrees (left hand and weight are down toward the floor).

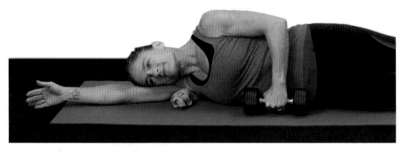

2. Keeping your left upper arm tucked against your side, rotate your forearm up and out, away from your stomach, until it's parallel to the floor and level with your left shoulder.

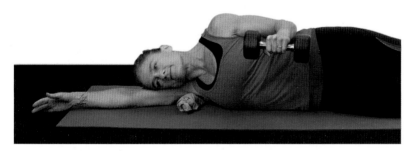

Lower your forearm slowly back to the starting position.

Switch arms and repeat.

Tennis Backhand with Resistance Tube

Do this exercise slowly and carefully, with good shoulders-back posture and with minimal weight to avoid straining the muscles. STOP if any pain occurs.

1. Anchor a resistance tube on a door or other immovable object on your left. Stand with good posture, feet shoulder-width apart, and grab the handle of the resistance tube with your right hand. Keeping your right upper arm close to your side, bend your right elbow 90 degrees, with your forearm pointing to the left, resting across your belly. Your left arm is relaxed at your side.

2. Exhale as you pull the tube away from your belly, keeping your upper arm close against your side and pivoting your hand and forearm to the right against resistance.

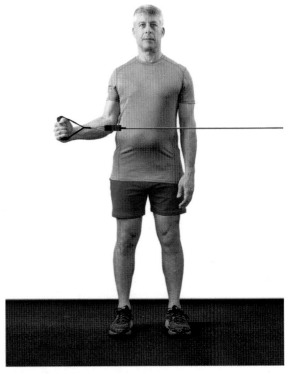

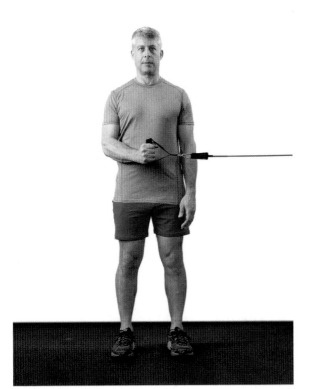

Inhale and slowly return to starting position.

Switch arms and repeat.

Tennis Forehand with Weights

Do this exercise slowly and carefully, with good shoulders-back posture and with minimal weight to avoid straining the muscles. STOP if any pain occurs.

1. Lie on your right side with your left arm resting along the left side of your body. Rest your head on a folded towel, if you like. Bend your right elbow 90 degrees and keep your right forearm on the floor extended straight out and perpendicular to your body. Hold a weight in your right hand with your palm up and wrist straight.

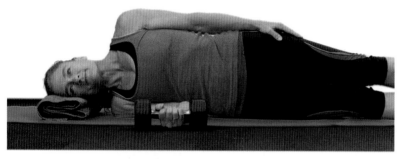

2. Exhale, and keeping the right upper arm tucked against your chest, rotate the forearm and hand up until it rests on your belly.

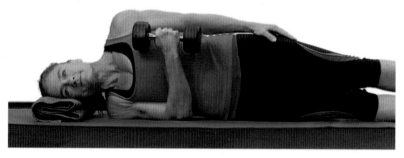

Inhale and lower the forearm slowly back to starting position.

Switch arms and repeat.

Tennis Forehand with Resistance Tube

Do this exercise slowly and carefully, with good shoulders-back posture and with minimal weight to avoid straining the muscles. STOP if any pain occurs.

1. Anchor a resistance tube on a door or other immovable object on your left. Stand with good posture, feet shoulder-width apart, and grab the handle of the resistance tube with your left hand. Keep your left upper arm close to the side, and bend your elbow to 90 degrees; your forearm should be pointing straight ahead with its palm facing to the right. Right arm is relaxed at its side.

2. Exhale as you pivot your forearm to the right across your belly against resistance, keeping the upper arm close against your side.

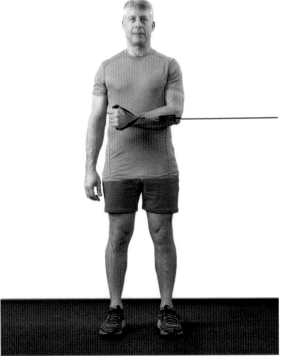

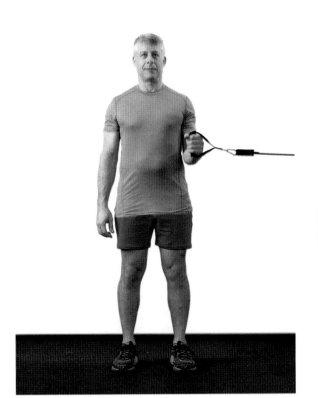

Inhale and return slowly to starting position.

Switch arms and repeat.

Thumbs Up with Weights

Do this exercise slowly and carefully, with good shoulders-back posture and with minimal weight to avoid straining the muscles. STOP if any pain occurs.

1. Stand with good posture feet shoulder-width apart, and hold a dumbbell in your right hand. Let both arms hang straight down at your sides.

2. Exhale and, keeping your arm straight and your thumb facing up, raise your right arm up at a 45-degree angle away from your body—midway between straight to the side and straight to the front (called the scaption plane). Start slowly and don't lift the dumbbell higher than the level of your shoulder.

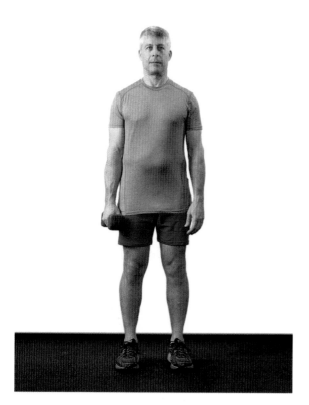

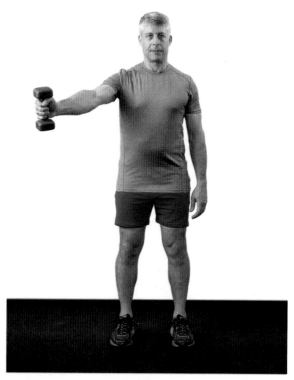

Inhale and slowly return to starting position.

Switch hands and repeat.

Thumbs Up with Resistance Tube

Do this exercise slowly and carefully, with good shoulders-back posture and with minimal weight to avoid straining the muscles. STOP if any pain occurs.

1. Stand with good posture, feet shoulder-width apart. Place the resistance tube under both feet and grab one end in your left hand for extra anchoring, if needed. Hold the other handle in your right hand.

2. Exhale and, keeping your arm straight and your thumb facing up, raise your right arm up at a 45-degree angle away from your body—midway between straight to the side and straight to the front (called the scaption plane). Start slowly and don't lift the tubing higher than the level of your shoulder.

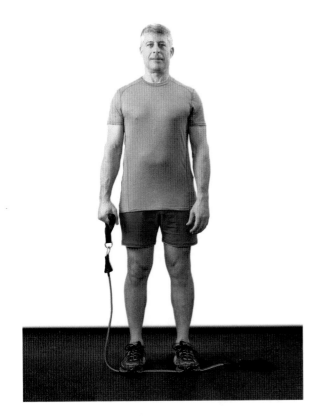

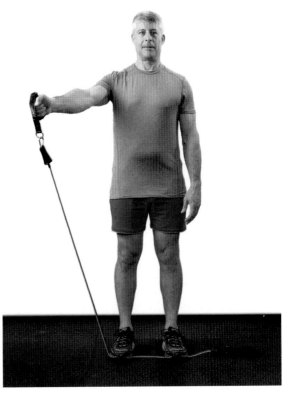

Inhale and slowly return to starting position.

Switch hands and repeat.

Chest Press with Weights

1. Lie on your back with knees bent and feet flat on the floor. Hold a dumbbell in each hand, keeping the upper arms close to your sides, elbows bent 90 degrees, fists pointing straight up, and palms facing your feet.

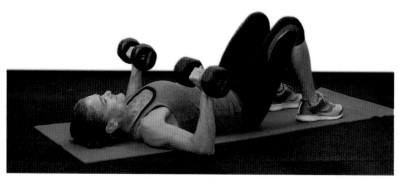

2. Exhale and, using your chest muscles, straighten your arms toward the ceiling. Finish with your arms directly over your shoulders, stopping just short of locking your elbows fully. Keep your lower back relaxed and flat on the floor.

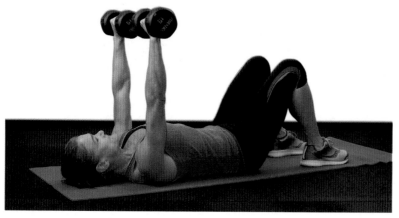

Inhale as you slowly bring the weights back down to starting position.

Standing Chest Press with Resistance Tube

1. Anchor a resistance tube on a doorknob or other immovable object of similar height behind you. Stand with good posture and step one foot forward about two feet into a staggered, stable stance. Grab a handle with each hand and bend both elbows, keeping your arms close to your sides, hands just in front of your chest, and palms down.

2. Exhale and press both arms forward until fully extended while simultaneously engaging your core by tightening your abdominal muscles.

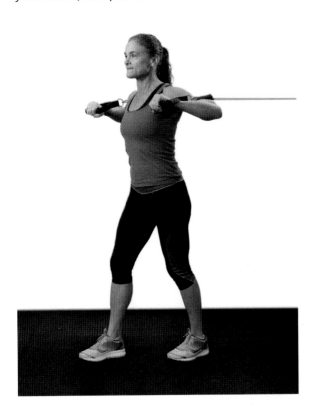

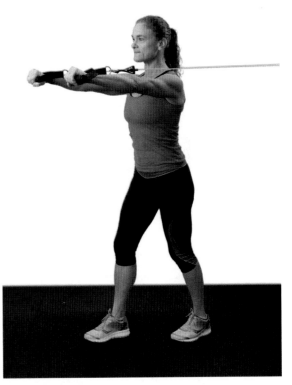

Inhale and slowly return to starting position.

Chest Fly with Weights

1. Lie on your back with knees bent and feet flat on the floor. Hold a dumbbell in each hand with your arms extended perpendicular to your body and palms facing upward.

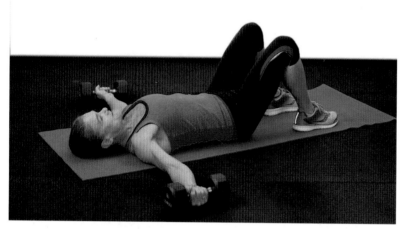

2. Exhale and, feeling your chest muscles engage, bend your elbows slightly as you raise your arms up toward each other to a point directly over the center of your chest. (Imagine you're hugging a large tree.) Don't lock your elbows.

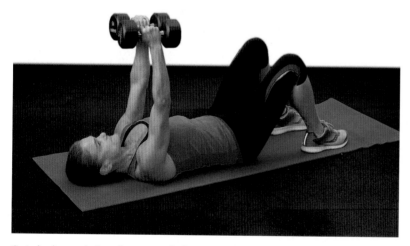

3. Inhale and simultaneously lower both arms to the sides, stopping just before your upper arms touch the floor.

Chest Fly with Resistance Tube

1. Anchor a resistance tube on a doorknob or other immovable object of similar height behind you. Stand with good posture and step one foot forward about two feet into a staggered, stable stance. Grab a handle with each hand, arms out to the sides just below shoulder height, with a slight bend in your elbows and palms facing inward.

2. Engage your core by tightening your abdominal muscles. Exhale and, feeling your chest muscles engage, bring your arms forward to a point in front of the center of your chest. (Imagine you're hugging a large tree.) Don't lock your elbows.

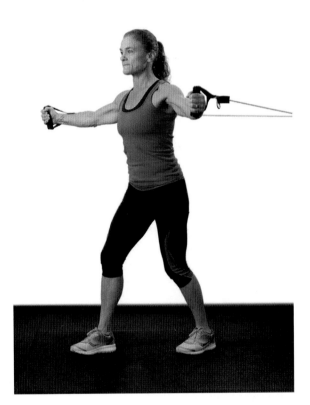

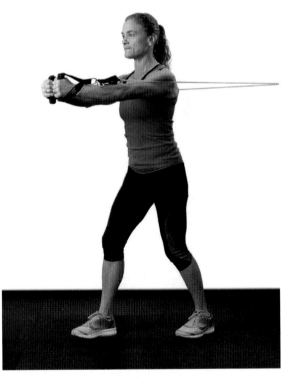

Inhale and slowly return to starting position.

73

Reverse Fly with Weights

This exercise is important for the posture of the upper body but can be straining. Start with just your body weight, and progress to wrist weights and light dumbbells as you get stronger. A small rolled-up towel or flat pillow placed under your pelvic bones/lower abdomen will flatten the lower back and may prove more comfortable.

1. Lie face down on the floor, keeping the back of your neck elongated. Rest your forehead on a small towel on the floor if more comfortable. Hold a dumbbell in each hand with your arms perpendicular to your body, elbows bent 90 degrees, and forearms and palms facing down.

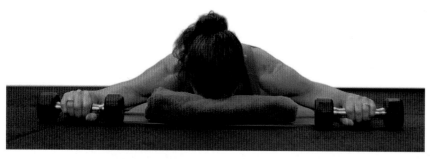

2. Exhale and, as you squeeze your shoulder blades together, lift your arms, hands, and dumbbells off the floor as a unit but no higher than shoulder height—you're only lifting the arms a couple of inches off the floor.

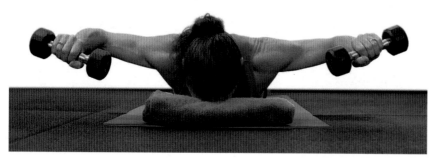

Inhale and slowly lower your arms back to starting position.

Seated Row with Resistance Tube

This exercise can also be done while sitting on an armless chair.

1. Sit on the floor with your legs extended (you may bend your knees slightly if needed). Loop the resistance tube around the middle of your feet or around an immovable, sturdy object in front of you. Extend your arms and grab the handles, holding them with your palms facing each other.

2. Exhale and, as you pinch your shoulder blades together and keep your shoulders back, pull the handles toward your armpits. Keep your arms tucked close to your sides.

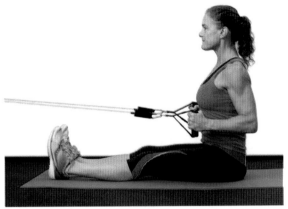

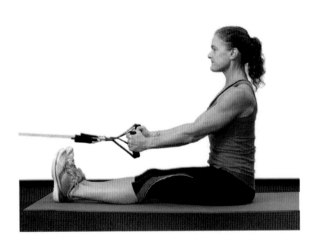

Inhale and slowly straighten your arms back to starting position.

Single-Arm Row with Weights

1. Standing with good posture, bend forward from the hips about 45 degrees. Keeping your lower and upper back straight, bring your left leg back a couple of feet to a stable position and slightly bend both knees. Place the palm of your right hand onto a chair back or counter for support. Holding a dumbbell in your left hand, let your left arm hang straight down from the shoulder. Engage your core by tightening your abdominal and lower back muscles.

2. Exhale and, without twisting your trunk, bring the dumbbell to your left shoulder, keeping your arm close to your side and your elbow pointing straight back behind you.

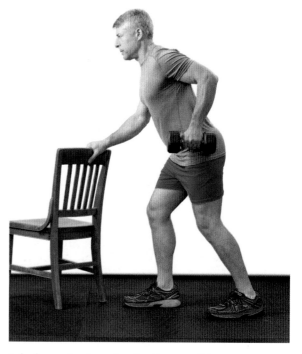

Inhale and return to starting position.

Switch sides and repeat.

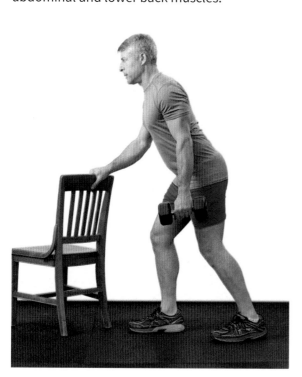

Biceps Curl with Weights

Biceps curls are isolation exercises as they mostly work a single muscle and joint. If you're going to do them, do them last after compound exercises. This exercise can be done while sitting.

1. Stand with good posture, feet shoulder-width apart. Hold a dumbbell in each hand, with your arms relaxed at your sides and palms facing forward.

2. Exhale and, engaging your core and keeping your elbows tucked against your sides, bend your elbows and bring both hands toward your relaxed shoulders. Don't arch your back. You can also alternate one arm at a time.

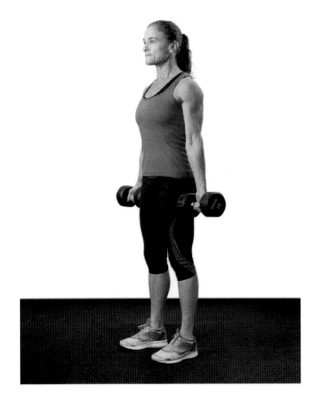
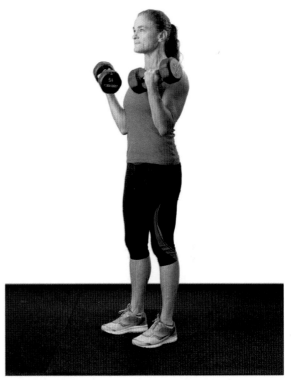

Inhale and slowly lower your hands to starting position.

Biceps Curl with Resistance Tube

Biceps curls are isolation exercises as they mostly work a single muscle and joint. If you're going to do them, do them last after compound exercises.

1. Stand with good posture, feet shoulder-width apart. Stand in the center of the resistance tube and grab a handle in each hand, arms relaxed at your sides and palms facing forward.

2. Exhale and, engaging your core and keeping your elbows tucked against your sides, bend your elbows and bring both hands toward your relaxed shoulders against the resistance. Don't arch your back. You can also alternate one arm at a time.

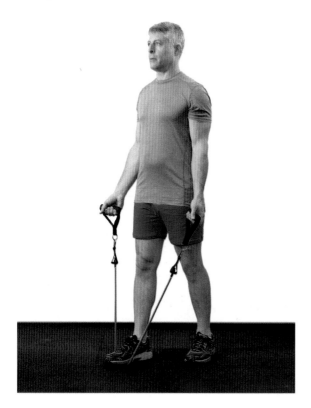

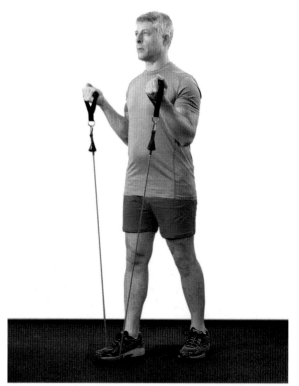

Inhale and slowly lower your hands to starting position.

Bent-Over Triceps Kick-Backs with Weights

Triceps extensions are isolation exercises as they mostly work a single muscle and joint. If you're going to do them, do them last after compound exercises.

1. Stand with good posture, feet shoulder-width apart, and bend forward from the hips about 45 degrees. Keeping your lower and upper back straight, bring your right leg back about two feet to a stable position and maintain a slight bend in both knees. Hold a dumbbell in your right hand and bend your elbow until your upper arm is parallel to the floor, your fist points down to the floor, and your palm faces in. Place the palm of your left hand onto a chair back or counter for support. Engage your core by tightening your abdominal and lower back muscles.

2. Exhale and, keeping your right upper arm still and tucked against your trunk, straighten your right elbow, bringing the dumbbell back until the entire arm is parallel to the floor. Stop short of locking your elbow.

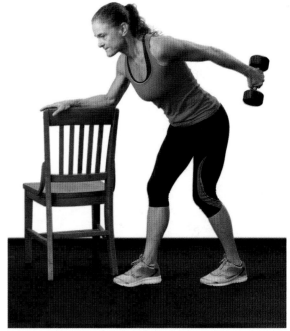

Inhale and return to starting position.

Switch arms and repeat.

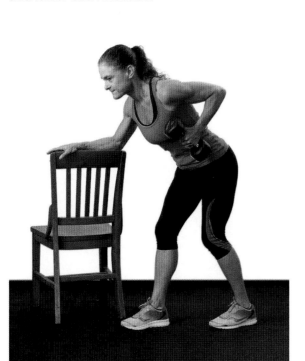

Standing Triceps Kick-Backs with Resistance Tubes

Triceps extensions are isolation exercises as they mostly work a single muscle and joint. If you're going to do them, do them last after compound exercises.

1. Anchor a resistance tube high on a door or other immovable object of similar height in front of you. Stand with good posture, feet shoulder-width apart or staggered for stability. Grab a handle in each hand, with elbows bent 90 degrees, palms facing in, and upper arms tucked tight against your sides. Engage your core by keeping your abdominal and lower back muscles tight.

2. Exhale and, using just your arms (not your body weight), push the tubes straight down, fully extending your arms but stopping short of locking your elbows. You can also alternate one arm at a time.

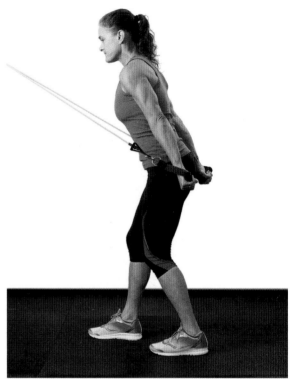

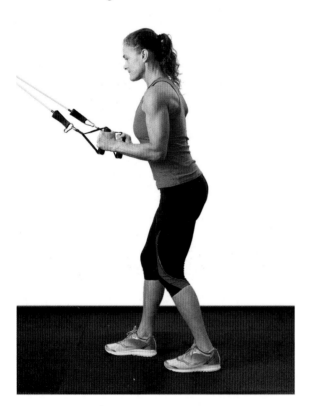

Inhale and slowly return your arms to starting position.

Core

These exercises work many muscles at once in the core and lower back area, including the abdominals, multifidus, and erector spinae.

Curl-Up with Weights

1. Lie on your back, feet flat on the floor with knees bent. Hold a medicine ball or dumbbell in front of your chest.

2. Exhale and engage your stomach muscles as you lift just your shoulders and the top of your upper back off the floor. Keep the back of your neck elongated.

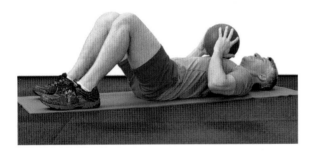

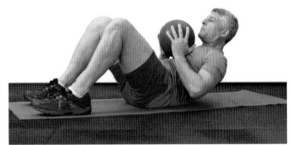

Inhale and slowly return to starting position.

Obliques Variation: To target the external obliques more, come up off the floor and slightly angle one shoulder toward the opposite side (lifting one up a little higher). Return to starting position and then lift and angle toward the other side.

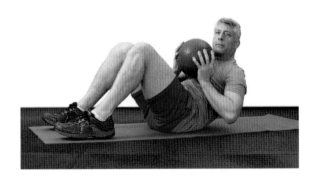

Trunk Rotation with Resistance Tube

This exercise can also be done with a medicine ball. Just hold the ball in your outstretched arms and do the same movements. If either version proves too difficult, bend your elbows to bring the resistance tubing or medicine ball closer to your body, which will put less stress on your core.

1. Anchor a resistance tube on a door or other immovable object at chest height off to your right side. Grab the tube handle(s) with your right hand and place your left hand on top of your right hand. Stand in an athletic posture with your legs shoulder-width apart and crouched at the knees and hips. Your upper body should be turned to the right—toward the anchor point—and both arms extended.

2. Exhale and, engaging your core by tightening your abdominal muscles, twist your trunk to the left against the resistance. Keep your shoulders back and the distance of your arms in front of your chest the same throughout the movement. Stop when your upper body and lower body are aligned, or your upper body is turned slightly farther to the left.

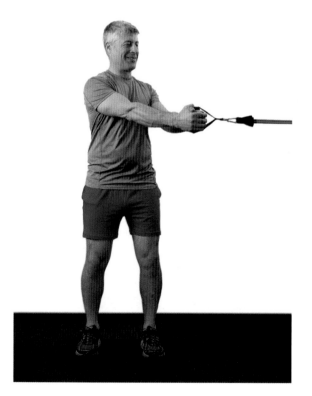

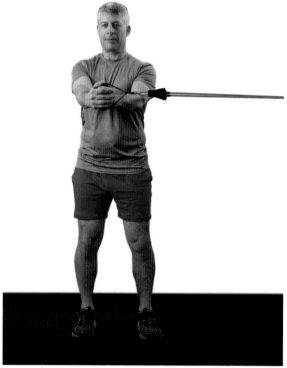

Inhale and slowly return to starting position.

Switch sides and repeat.

Bird Dog with Weights

This lower-back/core-strengthening exercise is a good place to start as a beginner. If it still proves to be difficult, just extend your arms without your legs, or skip the weights until you get stronger.

1. With weights on your ankles and wrists, assume a tabletop position on your hands and knees, keeping your hands below your shoulders and knees beneath your hips. Tighten your abdominals, pulling them up slightly and flattening your lower back.

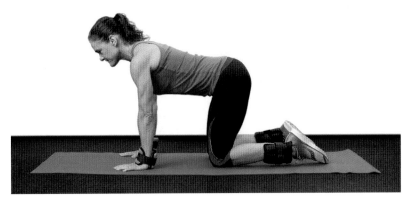

2. Exhale and extend your right arm straight out in front of you while simultaneously extending your left leg straight out behind you. Keep both limbs parallel to the ground.

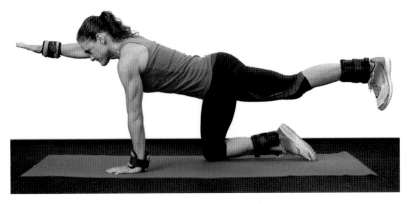

Inhale and return to starting position.

Repeat on the other side with your left arm and right leg.

Prone Extension with Weights

These prone extensions get progressively harder from A to D. Start with the single arm and advance as you get stronger. Use a rolled towel under your hips if it's more comfortable. Add wrist and ankle weights as you get stronger.

A. Single Arm

1. Lie face down, arms and legs outstretched (like Superman flying) and resting on the floor, parallel to each other.

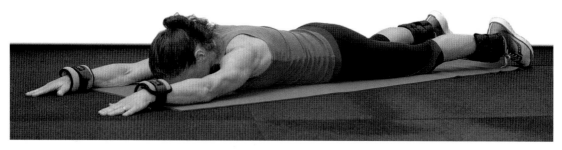

2. Exhale as you raise your right arm off the floor a few inches, without causing your trunk to twist.

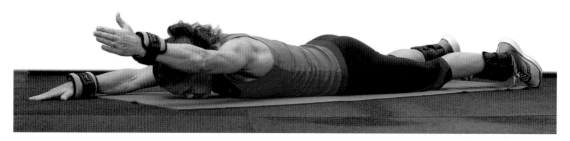

Inhale and slowly lower your arm to starting position.

Switch sides and repeat.

B. Single Leg

1. Lie face down, arms and legs outstretched (like Superman flying) and resting on the floor, parallel to each other.

2. Exhale as you raise your right leg off the floor a few inches, without causing your trunk to twist.

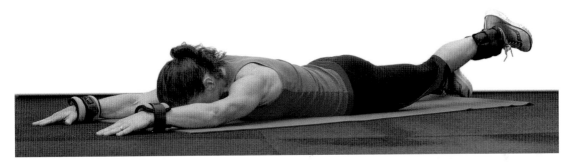

Inhale and slowly lower your leg to starting position.

Switch sides and repeat.

C. Opposite Arm and Leg

1. Lie face down, arms and legs outstretched (like Superman flying) and resting on the floor, parallel to each other.

2. Exhale as you raise your right arm and left leg off the floor a few inches, without causing your trunk to twist.

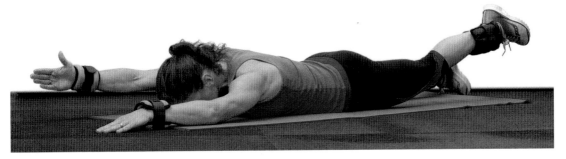

Inhale and slowly lower your arm and leg to starting position.

Repeat with your left arm and right leg.

D. Arms and Legs

1. Lie face down, arms and legs outstretched (like Superman flying) and resting on the floor, parallel to each other.

2. Exhale as you raise both arms and legs off the floor a few inches, without causing your trunk to twist.

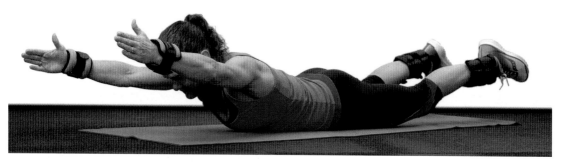

Inhale and slowly lower your arms and legs to starting position.

Lower Body

These lower-body exercises work many muscles at once in the lower body, including the glutes, hamstrings, quadriceps, gastrocnemius, and tibialis anterior.

Quad Setting

Strengthening the quadriceps muscles is very important for knee health. It's also an effective way to treat knee osteoarthritis as well as sarcopenia. Quad setting is a very gentle, isometric way of strengthening the quadriceps muscles. While limited in its ability to strengthen, this exercise is usually well-tolerated by problem knees, so it is a good place to start.

1. Sit or lie on the floor with your legs straight out in front of you. Place a rolled-up towel or pillow under your left knee.

2. Exhale and, as you pull your left toes back, press the back of your left knee down on the towel. Feel the front of your left thigh muscles tighten as you press down.

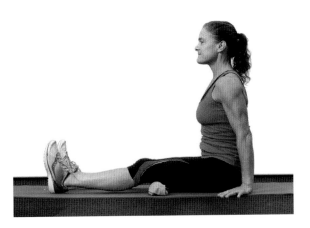

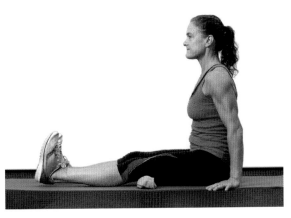

Hold for 10 to 12 seconds, then relax.

Switch sides and repeat.

Repeat as often as is comfortable, building up the intensity by pushing harder as your strength improves.

Seated Leg Raise with Weights

1. Sit in a chair with ankle weights on and straighten your left leg in front of you so it's parallel to the ground.

2. Exhale and, keeping your left leg straight, lift it a little higher—attempting to lift the back of the thigh off the chair seat without leaning your body backward.

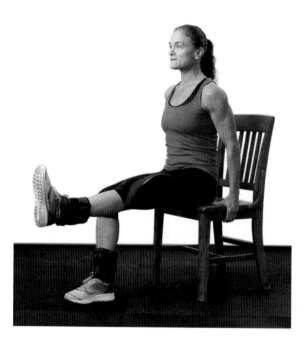

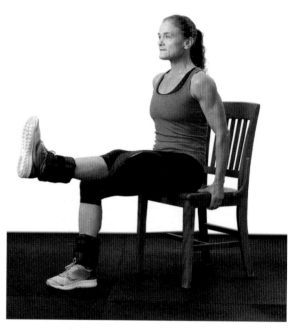

Inhale and lower to starting position.

Switch sides and repeat.

To strengthen other parts of the quadriceps muscle, turn the foot slightly toward the outside or inside as you exhale and lift the leg off the chair.

Leg Press with Resistance Tube

1. Sit in a sturdy chair. Wrap the resistance tube around your right foot, crossing it once between your foot and your hands for safety, and grasp the handles in your hands. Inhale and bend your right knee to bring it closer to your body. Remove any slack and increase the tension in the tube.

2. Exhale and straighten your right leg against the resistance. Stop short of locking your knee.

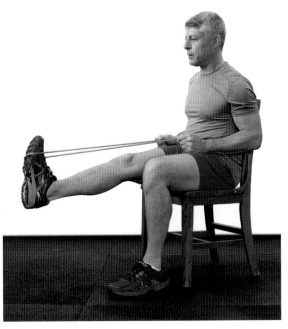

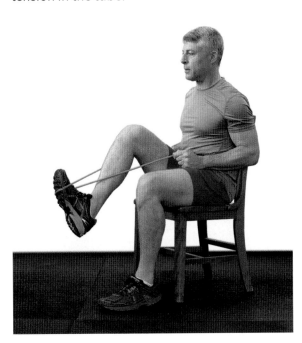

Inhale and slowly return the knee to its bent position.

Switch sides and repeat.

Standing Leg Curl with Weights

1. Put on ankle weights and stand with good posture, legs close together. Face a counter or chair back and hold on for support.

2. Exhale and bend your left knee to bring your left heel toward your butt. Stop when your left shin is about parallel to the floor.

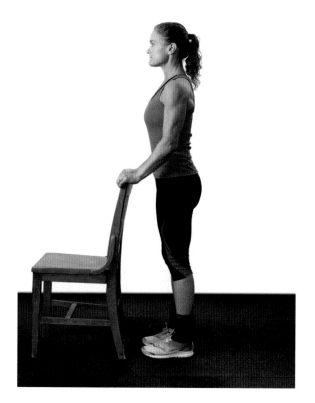

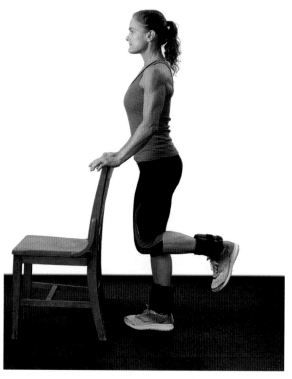

Inhale and slowly return to starting position.

Switch sides and repeat.

Prone Leg Curl with Resistance Tube

A small rolled-up towel or flat pillow placed under your pelvic bones/lower abdomen will flatten the lower back and may prove more comfortable.

1. Anchor a resistance tube to a door or other immovable object behind you. Loop the tube around your right ankle. Lie face down and rest your forehead on your crossed hands, which should be placed in front of you on the floor.

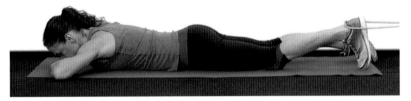

2. Exhale and bend your right knee to bring your right heel toward your butt against the resistance. Stop when your right shin is perpendicular to the floor.

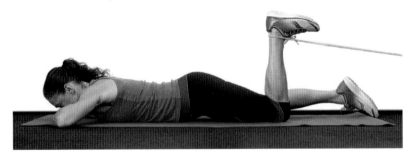

Inhale and slowly return to starting position.

Switch sides and repeat.

Chair Squat with Weights

Chair squats are a little easier than regular squats, and give an added dose of safety if balance is an issue. This can also be done with a medicine ball.

1. Sit on the front half of a sturdy chair with both feet flat on the floor. Hold a dumbbell in each hand with your arms crossed at the wrists and close to your chest.

2. Exhale and, leaning slightly forward, rise from the chair while keeping your arms in place. Keep your back straight and don't let your knees collapse inward or extend beyond the level of your toes.

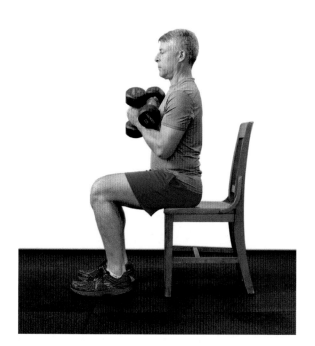

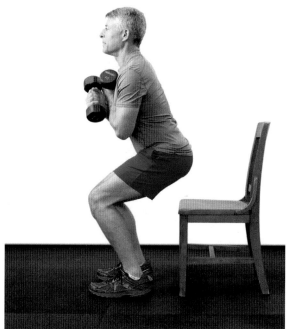

Inhale as you lower yourself back down to a seated position.

Chair Squat with Resistance Tube

Easier than regular squats, chair squats give an added dose of safety if balance is an issue.

1. Sit on the front half of a sturdy chair with both feet flat on the floor. Place the center of a resistance tube beneath your feet. Extend your arms down, toward the outsides of your knees, and grasp the handles. Remove any slack from the tubing to create some resistance.

2. Exhale and, leaning slightly forward, rise from the chair against the resistance, keeping your arms extended. Keep your back straight and don't let your knees collapse inward or extend beyond the level of your toes.

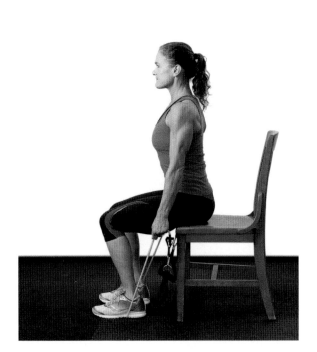

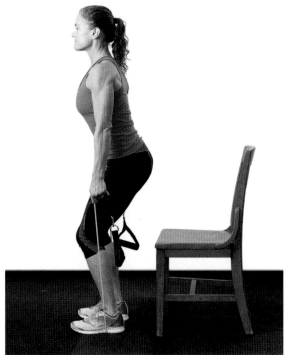

Inhale as you slowly lower yourself back down to a seated position.

Squat with Weights

This exercise can also be done with a medicine ball.

1. Stand with your feet hip-width apart and slightly flared out. Hold two dumbbells with your arms hanging down loosely, or crossed at the wrists and close to your chest.

2. Inhale and slowly bend your hips and knees as if to sit down in a chair, keeping your back straight and your weight toward your heels. Don't allow your knees to extend forward past your toes or let them collapse to the inside. Keep them pressed out during the entire movement—squatting down and standing back up.

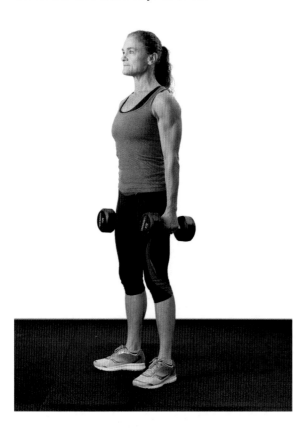

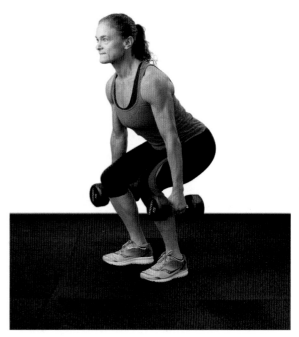

Lower yourself until your thighs are parallel or lower to the ground.

Exhale as you raise yourself back up to a standing position.

Squat with Resistance Tube

1. Place the center of the resistance tube beneath your feet. Stand with your feet hip-width apart and slightly flared out. Extend your arms toward the floor and squat down, bending your knees and hips until your thighs are parallel or lower to the ground. Grasp the tube handles and remove any slack to create some resistance.

2. Exhale and, keeping your arms extended, slowly rise to a standing position against resistance. Keep your back straight and your weight toward your heels. Don't allow your knees to extend forward past your toes or let them collapse to the inside—keep them pressed out during the entire standing up and squatting down movement.

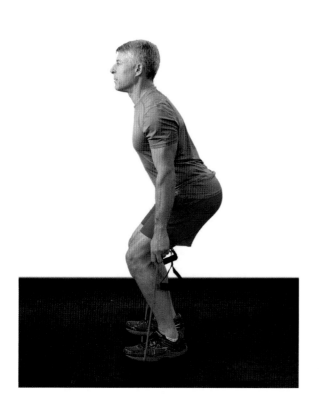

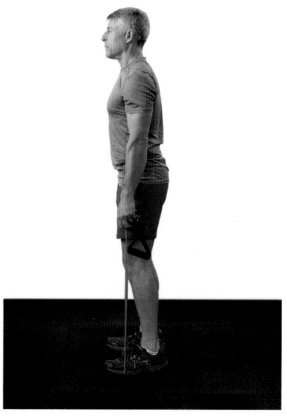

Lower yourself back down until your thighs are parallel or lower to the ground.

Seated Leg Extension with Weights

This exercise can also be done on a regular chair with a firm pillow under the exercising thigh to elevate your foot off the floor.

1-2. Sit in a tall chair with ankle weights on both legs. Exhale as you slowly extend your left leg in front of you. Stop short of locking the knee.

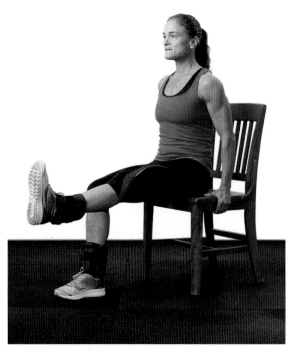

Inhale and slowly lower the leg.

Switch sides and repeat.

Seated Leg Extension with Resistance Tube

This exercise can also be done on a regular-height chair with a firm pillow under the exercising thigh to elevate your foot off the floor.

1. Attach a resistance tube to a back leg of a tall chair or the lower part of a door or other immovable, sturdy object behind the chair. Sit in the chair and loop the tube around your left ankle and foot.

2. Exhale as you slowly extend your left leg in front of you. Stop short of locking the knee.

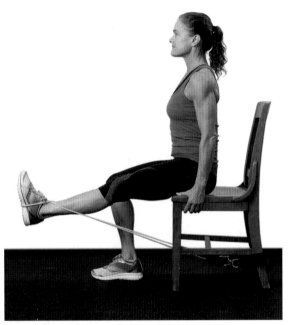

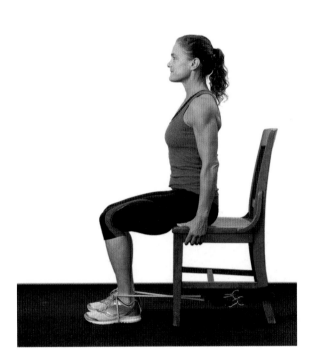

Inhale and slowly lower the leg.

Switch sides and repeat.

Heel Raise with Weights

1. Stand with good posture, feet hip-width apart. Hold a dumbbell in each hand, arms relaxed at your sides.

2. Exhale and slowly raise your heels off the floor, coming up onto the balls of your feet.

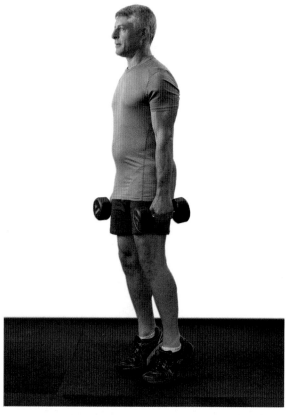

Inhale and slowly lower your heels to the floor.

Heel Raise with Resistance Tube

1. Place the center of the resistance tube beneath the balls of both feet. Grab the handles of the tube and stand with good posture with your feet hip-width apart. Slide your hands upward, along the sides of your body, to remove any slack and create more resistance.

2. Exhale and, while maintaining resistance, slowly raise your heels off the floor, coming up onto the balls of your feet.

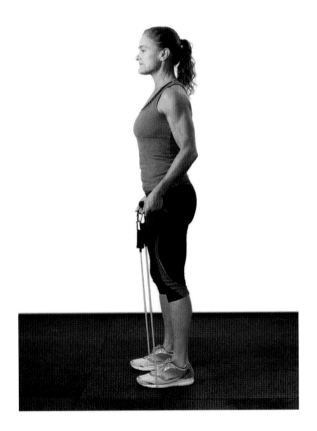

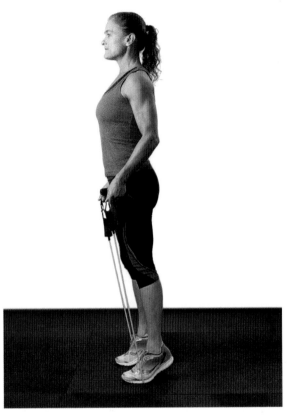

Inhale and slowly lower your heels to the floor.

CHAPTER 6

Sarcopenia and Diet

"If we could give every individual the right amount of nourishment and exercise, not too little and not too much, we would have found the safest way to health."

—Hippocrates

Older Adults and Protein Deficits

Diet and nutrition play an enormous role in healthy living, and unique challenges as we age make nutritional considerations even more important. In fact, insufficient protein intake appears to be the biggest dietary issue when it comes to sarcopenia and aging. As a 2013 *Journal of the American Medical Directors Association* study illustrates, 15 to 38 percent of older men and 27 to 41 percent of older women ingest less than the recommended daily allowance (RDA) for protein. At the very least, sarcopenic individuals need to bump up their protein intake to the recommended levels unless otherwise directed by a medical professional.

When you consider that many experts believe that even older adults without sarcopenia should exceed the RDA of protein, the percentage of older adults not consuming adequate amounts grows even larger.

It's not always clear why older adults consume less protein. Some theories are:

> Diets that limit calories or protein consumption.

> Lack of desire to cook for oneself.

> Decreased ability to smell or taste, making food less desirable.

> Decreased appetite, sometimes due to the side effects of medications.

> Depression and isolation, which can remove the social aspects of eating.

> Chronic illnesses causing GI upset, bowel difficulties, or nausea.

> Residential and nursing home environments resulting in an inability to choose what and when to eat, insufficient or unappetizing food, resistance to eating in a dining hall setting, and being removed from the other aspects of food, like the preparation process.

Consuming inadequate amounts of protein is just one part of the problem. Older bodies can have difficulty utilizing dietary protein while also requiring more protein. In the balance of building up muscles (a result of anabolism, a constructive process) versus losing muscles (a result of catabolism, a destructive process), the protein deficit tips the balance toward catabolism, or losing muscle tissue. Science has offered several age-related physiologic phenomena to explain how protein factors play a role in this process:

> Reduced bioavailability of dietary amino acids—the building blocks of protein—possibly due to changes in the absorption in the gut and liver.

> Declining anabolic response to protein ingestion. As we age, the normal build-up of muscle proteins in response to food becomes blunted, likely the result of a change in the response to the body's own hormones.

> Reduced synthesis of anabolic hormones. Hormones within the body stimulate muscle growth, so as these hormones decrease with age, so does muscle growth.

> Increase in inflammatory conditions. The chronic low-grade inflammation that appears to be associated with the aging body may also both inhibit the synthesis and promote the breakdown of muscle proteins, contributing to sarcopenia.

> Diminished physical activity level. The anabolic effects of amino acids appear to be enhanced by physical activity and impaired by a sedentary lifestyle.

> Coexisting acute and chronic diseases. Acute illnesses—especially with associated vomiting or diarrhea—and chronic conditions like cancer can both decrease the bioavailability of, and increase the requirement for, proteins.

Most researchers agree that increasing the amount of protein in the diet stimulates the synthesis of muscle proteins. And since compared to younger people, older people require a higher intake of protein for muscle protein synthesis, increasing protein will in turn lead to more muscle mass and strength, and lessen the deleterious effects of sarcopenia. While adding more protein to the diet has not been shown to have negative effects for the kidneys or other organs in healthy older adults, it's still a good idea to consult your physician regarding any significant dietary changes, especially if you have medical problems.

How Much More Protein Should You Eat?

The European Society for Clinical Nutrition and Metabolism and the European Union Geriatric Medicine Society—who appointed an international study group (called the PROT-AGE study group) to review dietary protein requirements—came up with the following evidence-based recommendations for protein consumption for people over 65 years old:

> 1.0–1.2 grams (g) of protein per kilogram (kg) of body weight, per day, for healthy older people.

> 1.2–1.5 grams of protein per kg of body weight, per day, if physically active—both for endurance- and resistance-type exercises

> People with acute and chronic diseases may need even more protein, although those with kidney disease but not on dialysis may need less, so seek medical advice first.

To calculate your requirements, multiply your body weight in pounds by .45 to get your weight in kilograms. Then multiply that by the number of grams of protein you should be eating.

> **Example 1:** A 125-pound person = 57kg. A 65+-year-old adult who weighs this much would have a baseline protein intake requirement of 57–68 g per day.

   If engaged in PRE, their protein intake requirement should increase to 68–86g per day.

> **Example 2:** A 150-pound person = 68kg. A 65+-year-old adult who weighs this much would have a baseline protein intake requirement of 68–82g per day.

If engaged in PRE, their protein intake requirement should increase to 82–102g per day.

> **Example 3:** A 175-pound person = 79kg. A 65+-year-old adult who weighs this much would have a baseline protein intake requirement of 79–95g per day.

If engaged in PRE, their protein intake requirement should increase to 95–119g per day.

Following is a table of the approximate protein content of various foods. To figure out serving sizes, you can use a kitchen scale or you can eyeball it. Three ounces of cooked meat is about the size of the palm of the hand or a bar of bath soap. Three ounces of cooked seafood is a little larger, about the size of a checkbook. Half a cup of legumes and grains is about the size of your closed fist. And 1 ounce of nuts is a small handful.

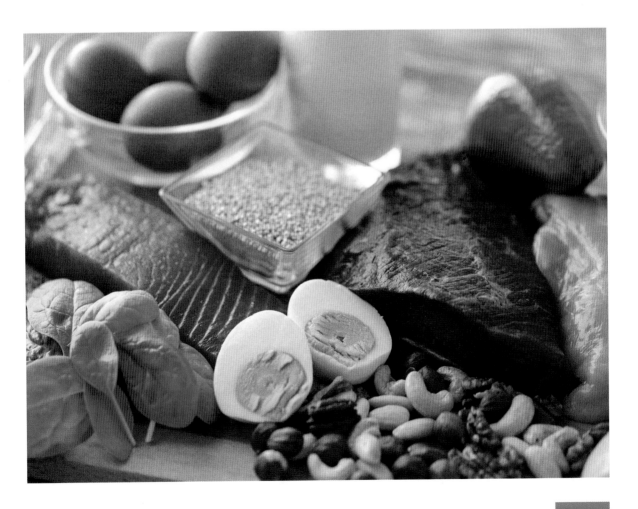

Protein in Various Foods

	FOOD (COOKED)	SERVING SIZE	CALORIES	PROTEIN
MEAT, POULTRY, EGGS	Chicken, skinless breast	3 ounces	142	27g
	Chicken, skinless dark meat	3 ounces	178	22g
	Egg	1 large egg	71	6g
	Ham	3 ounces	139	14g
	Lamb	3 ounces	172	23g
	Pork	3 ounces	122	23g
	Steak	3 ounces	158	26g
	Turkey, skinless breast	3 ounces	137	25g
	Turkey, skinless dark meat	3 ounces	163	24g
SEAFOOD	Halibut	3 ounces	94	19g
	Lobster	3 ounces	76	16g
	Salmon	3 ounces	155	22g
	Scallops	3 ounces	75	14g
	Shrimp	3 ounces	101	20g
	Trout	3 ounces	162	23g
	Tuna	3 ounces	99	22g
LEGUMES, GRAINS, VEGETABLES	Adzuki beans	½ cup	147	9g
	Black beans	½ cup	114	8g
	Black-eyed peas	½ cup	100	7g
	Chickpeas	½ cup	134	7g
	Edamame	½ cup	95	9g
	Fava beans	½ cup	94	7g
	Kidney beans, red	½ cup	112	8g
	Lentils	½ cup	101	9g
	Lima beans	½ cup	105	6g
	Peas, green	½ cup	59	4g
	Pinto beans	½ cup	197	11g
	Quinoa	½ cup	111	4g
	Spinach, cooked	½ cup	41	3g
	Tempeh	½ cup	160	15g
	Tofu, firm	½ cup	94	10g
	Wheat berries	½ cup	151	6g

	FOOD (COOKED)	SERVING SIZE	CALORIES	PROTEIN
NUTS AND SEEDS	Almonds	1 ounce	163	6g
	Cashews	1 ounce	162	4g
	Chia seeds	1 ounce	138	5g
	Flax seeds	1 ounce	140	6g
	Peanut butter, creamy natural	1 tablespoon	95	4g
	Peanuts	1 ounce	166	7g
	Pistachios	1 ounce	161	6g
	Pumpkin seeds	1 ounce	159	9g
	Soy nuts	1 ounce	120	12g
	Sunflower seeds	1 ounce	140	6g
	Walnuts	1 ounce	185	4g
DAIRY PRODUCTS	Cottage cheese, 1% fat	4 ounces	81	14g
	Milk, cow's, skim	1 cup	86	8g
	Milk, goat's	1 cup	168	9g
	Milk, soy	1 cup	132	8g
	Mozzarella, part skim	1 ounce	72	7g
	String cheese, nonfat	1 piece, 0.75 ounce	50	6g
	Yogurt, Greek	6 ounces	100	18g
	Yogurt, regular, nonfat	1 cup	100	11g

Chart adapted from Learning Today's Dietician https://www.todaysdietitian.com/pdf/webinars/ProteinContentofFoods.pdf.

Types and Timing of Proteins

Proteins from animal sources are not the same as those from plant sources. While no definitive evidence yet exists as to which is better for older muscles, animal proteins may have an advantage. This is because animal proteins are complete proteins—they contain all the essential amino acids—and are more digestible. Vegetarians need to eat a larger and more varied amount of plant-based proteins because most plant-based proteins are incomplete, i.e., lack one of the nine essential amino acids.

When should you consume your daily recommended protein? While you can eat the largest percentage in one meal, it'd be a super-sized protein portion. Timing is also a factor when exercising as you want to ensure you have protein around physical activity so the working muscles have the raw materials they need to build. With these considerations in mind, most researchers agree that spreading proteins out evenly over all the day's meals works best. For the average older adult, this could mean consuming about 25 to 30 grams of high-quality protein at each of the day's three meals.

Dietary Recommendations and Tips

In addition to consuming too little protein, many diets of older adults are unvaried and limited in nutritional content. Following a Mediterranean-type diet rich in fruits, vegetables, skinless poultry, fish, limited red meat, and extra-virgin olive oil, and low in sweets and highly processed foods, is beneficial. Try to eat a variety of animal- and plant-sourced proteins, with eggs, dairy, beans, legumes, and grains making up the balance of the necessary proteins. I also recommend having sufficient quantities of anti-inflammatory foods in your diet, like blueberries, pineapples, walnuts, and green leafy vegetables.

Here are some ideas to get more protein into your meals:

Breakfast: Not just toast and tea. Add a hardboiled egg, peanut butter on toast, or a protein smoothie made with fruit, Greek yogurt, and seeds.

Lunch: Not just a green salad. Add tuna, some kidney beans or pumpkin seeds, or have Greek yogurt or peanut butter.

Dinner: This is usually easy as many people eat their meat or fish at this meal. Great vegetarian options are lentil soup or a three-bean salad with spinach and cheese.

If you need more ideas or would prefer a personalized approach, a consultation with a nutritionist or dietician can give you more direction.

Protein Supplementation

If you can't meet the protein nutritional requirements needed to reverse and prevent sarcopenia through food alone, supplementation is a practical and convenient alternative. Advantages are that they can be easily timed for between meals or around workout sessions, are complete proteins, and can be cost-effective. Some of the available sources, which come in a variety of forms and flavors, are:

> **Whey protein:** The most popular protein supplement, this is the by-product of cheese production and is easily digested. Whey protein is a "fast" protein because of its quick absorption in the gut, making it a great choice for after workouts when muscles are building. It contains all the essential amino acids, as well as branched-chain amino acids—chains of three essential amino acids common in skeletal muscle. Whey protein appears to be better retained than casein protein in older individuals.

> **Casein protein:** Derived from milk, casein is a "slow" protein because of a longer absorption time, creating a stream of protein for between meals or at bedtime.

> **Egg albumin protein:** Derived from egg whites, egg protein has a high essential amino acid content, and is great for those with milk allergies.

> **Other protein supplement sources:** You'll also find protein in soy, goat's milk, wheat, and peas.

> **Essential amino acid supplementation:** This is another popular choice; some studies have shown a benefit, especially from those containing leucine or its metabolite, and appears to also have an important role combating sarcopenia.

FORMS OF WHEY PROTEIN

The popular whey protein supplements come in three common forms, differing in how they are extracted and treated, which alters their ingredients and absorbability.

1. Whey concentrates are the most basic and cost-effective form, usually containing about 80 percent protein.
2. Whey isolates are the purest and most expensive form, typically about 92 percent pure, with many non-protein elements like lactose, fat, and cholesterol removed.
3. Whey hydrolysates are broken down for faster digestion.

Many studies have investigated the use of protein supplementation to combat sarcopenia with conflicting results. Some show improvement in physical function while others do not. An explanation of this discrepancy could be that the studies used different types of supplements or the baseline health status of the participants varied. Ultimately, protein supplementation for the prevention or treatment of sarcopenia does appear to be warranted, especially in cases where an older adult is chronically ill, healing from a trauma or surgery, appears weak or malnourished, is showing signs of cognitive or functional decline, and has difficulty consuming adequate amounts of protein-rich foods.

Older Adults and Frail, Elderly Adults

A 2016 study published in the *Journal of Nutrition* enrolled 60 healthy older adults, aged 56 to 66 years old, to drink either a milk-based protein supplement or a non-protein supplement at breakfast and lunch. After 24 weeks, lean tissue mass increased in the protein-supplement group by .45 kg, compared to a decrease of .16 kg in the control group. The researchers surmised that consuming a balanced, optimized amount of protein during meals might be effective in preserving lean tissue mass (muscles) in older adults.

What's significant about this case is that the study participants were healthy middle-aged and older adults, yet they still added muscle compared to participants who didn't supplement. But what about frail or much older subjects?

A 2012 study cited in the *Journal of the American Medical Directors Association* enrolled 65 frail elderly people and divided them into two groups. One group ingested 15g of protein supplementation at breakfast and lunch, while the other ingested a placebo supplement, for 24 weeks. While both groups had similar results when analyzing skeletal muscle mass and strength, only the protein-supplementation group had significant improvement in the Short Physical Battery test, the physical performance test that assesses balance, walking speed, and repeated standing up from a chair. The placebo group had no change. This is momentous because even a small increase in the score for this valid and reliable evaluation has been shown to reduce the risk of falling, losing independence, having longer hospital stays and re-admissions, and dying from all causes.

Finally, a systematic review evaluating the effect of high-protein oral nutritional supplements was published in *Ageing Research Reviews*. It included over 3,700 people with a mean age of 74. The 2012 review and analysis discovered reduced hospital re-admissions, reduced complications, and improved grip strength in the protein supplementation groups.

Synergistic Effects When Combining PRE and Supplements

With studies supporting the use of protein supplements to combat sarcopenia, a 2016 study in the *American Journal of Clinical Nutrition* evaluated what effects both supplementing protein and exercising would have on sarcopenia. The participants were 130 sarcopenic elderly people with a mean age of 80 years old. Everyone took part in a 12-week exercise program and approximately half supplemented with whey protein, essential amino acids—including leucine—and vitamin D, while the other group supplemented with placebos. The results showed that regular exercise combined with protein and vitamin supplements increased muscle mass and enhanced "other aspects that contribute to well-being in sarcopenic elderly."

***

The takeaway from these studies marries with the consensus of many experts on sarcopenia—increasing the intake of protein is a very important part of a treatment but should be done in conjunction with PRE to maximize benefits. This is analogous to an osteoporosis treatment and prevention protocol, where a diet or supplementation regimen should include bone-building minerals, but weight-bearing exercise designed to stress the bone is also needed for the bones to absorb those nutrients. The body needs to work—and be challenged—to take those raw materials and put them to use in order to get stronger and healthier.

Other Supplements

Developing a comprehensive nutrient regimen is important to improving and maintaining health. Following are some of the supplements that have been studied and shown promise in maintaining muscle strength, decreasing fractures, and combating other symptoms of sarcopenia.

Vitamin D

There has been growing evidence in the last decade that many older people have inadequate levels of vitamin D in their bodies. The National Health and Nutrition Examination Survey estimated the prevalence of vitamin D deficiency to be 41.6 percent. This figure may be low for seniors—some experts argue that these studies underestimate the problem because the required amounts for older adults to prevent chronic illnesses are even higher than those used to define deficiency.

Vitamin D deficiency plays a role in sarcopenia as well as chronic diseases like osteoporosis—and its resulting bone fractures. Vitamin D receptors are present in skeletal (and cardiac) muscle, which are centrally involved in building muscle mass and strength. This may explain why vitamin D supplementation can decrease falls and fall-induced fractures. Sufficient amounts of vitamin D appear to be an important component of preventing and treating sarcopenia and reducing osteoporotic fractures.

Omega-3s

Omega-3 polyunsaturated fatty acids are well-known anti-inflammatories that are beneficial for preventing mortality in patients at risk for coronary heart disease and ischemic stroke. While the results of studies on the effect of omega-3s on sarcopenia have been mixed, some studies have demonstrated their benefit to enhance the anabolic effects of insulin and amino acids to synthesize proteins, while others have linked their deficiency with decreased muscle function. Combined with adequate protein intake, vitamin D supplementation, and PRE exercise, omega-3s are a good bet.

Leucine

Leucine is a potent branched-chain amino acid, one of the nine essential amino acids important for protein synthesis. Leucine supplementation has shown promise in the treatment of sarcopenia, not only on its own, but also it may have additive effects when combined with protein, vitamin D, and omega-3s.

WHAT ABOUT TESTOSTERONE?

Testosterone is a strong anabolic steroid that gradually diminishes as men and women age. Supplemental testosterone has shown to have short-term benefits in some studies of healthy older men—including increased muscle mass and strength. But significant problems in one *New England Journal of Medicine* study—including adverse cardiovascular events—resulted in the early termination of the study for safety reasons. Unfortunately, as this study points out, there are serious questions about the long-term safety of testosterone supplements, and at this point they cannot be recommended.

***

Researchers are busy at work investigating other possible treatments for sarcopenia, including amino acid metabolites and safer versions of steroids. Anti-inflammatories and antioxidants also appear to play important roles in combating age-related stress. Much is at stake—sarcopenia is an extremely debilitating and costly problem in the United States and throughout the world.

CHAPTER 7

F-A-C-S Process: Sarcopenia Self-Tests

"Know thyself."

—Socrates

Knowing the risks of sarcopenia and being able to recognize its signs are important to taking steps to prevent it. An easy way to test yourself is via the Find-Assess-Confirm-Severity (F-A-C-S) process, which was designed by the European Working Group on Sarcopenia in Older People (EWGSOP) to create a uniform pathway for clinicians and researches to diagnose and classify sarcopenia. Use the self-tests in this chapter to assess yourself or an aging loved one. If you don't think you need the tests now, keep them handy for future use.

Find

While a physician's clinical suspicion is an effective way to find suspected sarcopenia cases, there's a simple, at-home self-reporting tool called the SARC-F questionnaire, which the EWGSOP recommends as a first step to find probable cases of sarcopenia.

This brief five-question survey attempts to ascertain one's feelings of weakness and need for assistance. Several studies have examined the effectiveness of the SARC-F screening test, and it has proven to be consistent and valid for detecting persons at risk.

SARC-F Questionnaire

1. Strength: How much difficulty do you have in lifting and carrying 10 pounds? (Examples of things weighing 10 pounds include: a three-month-old baby, a small dog, a vacuum cleaner, or holiday ham.)

❑ One = 0   ❑ Some = 1   ❑ A lot or unable = 2

2. Assistance in walking: How much difficulty do you have walking across a room?

❑ None = 0   ❑ Some = 1   ❑ A lot, unable, or use aids = 2

3. Rising from a chair: How much difficulty do you have transferring from a chair or bed?

❑ None = 0   ❑ Some = 1   ❑ A lot or unable without help = 2

4. Climbing stairs: How much difficulty do you have climbing a flight of 10 stairs?

❑ None = 0   ❑ Some = 1   ❑ A lot or unable = 2

5. Falls: How many times have you fallen in the past year?

❑ None = 0   ❑ 1–3 falls = 1   ❑ 4 or more falls = 2

Scores of 4 or more have been shown to correlate with more difficulty performing activities of daily living—cooking, cleaning, and dressing—with lower grip strength, lower knee extensor strength, a higher likelihood of recent hospitalizations, and increased mortality.

Assess

The chair stand and grip strength tests are physical tests that can be used to assess if low muscle strength is present. While testing grip strength is a simple procedure, it does require something called a hand-held dynamometer, and is usually performed in a more formal clinical setting. The chair stand (or rise) test, however, can easily be tried at home.

The Chair Stand, or Rise, Test

The chair stand, or rise, test assesses the quadriceps muscle strength—very important thigh muscles needed for standing, walking, balance, avoiding falls, and maintaining independence.

To Perform the Test:

1. Sit in the middle of a 17-inch-high seat of a sturdy armless chair with your feet flat on the floor. Crossing at the wrists, place your hands on opposite shoulders.

2. Now stand, keeping your back straight and your arms hugged tightly against your chest.

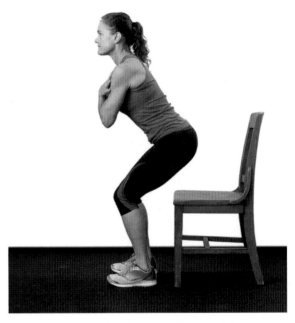

3. Once you reach a full standing position, immediately sit back down.

Time how long it takes you to rise and sit back down five times from a chair, without the assistance of the arms.

Reference Range:

A large study of healthy men and women aged 60 years and older determined that 8.5 seconds was the average time for completion, regardless of age or sex. Therefore, the more north of 9 seconds it takes to stand up five times, the weaker the leg muscles are.

Timed Chair Stand Test

An alternative to the chair stand test is the timed chair stand test, or the 30-second chair stand test, which measures the number of times a person can rise out of a chair to a full standing position and then sit back down again within 30 seconds. This test adds an endurance component but is still a convenient way to measure leg muscle strength.

Reference Range:

The numbers listed are the *below*-average scores. If you can stand from the chair the number of times listed, or more, for your given age and sex, your leg muscles are not deemed weak enough for concern.

AGE	MEN	WOMEN
60–64 years	<14	<12
65–69 years	<12	<11
70–74 years	<12	<10
75–79 years	<11	<10
80–84 years	<10	<9
85–89 years	<8	<8
90–94 years	<7	<4

If the SARC-F score is equal to or greater than 4, and the Chair Stand Test or Timed Chair Stand Test number is less than average, it's likely you have sarcopenia. You should begin treatment while confirming and assessing the severity.

Confirm

To confirm the suspected presence of sarcopenia, the EWGSOP then recommends testing with MRIs, CTs, or dual-energy absorptiometry (DXA) at research or clinical centers specializing in sarcopenia and its related disorders. A visit to your primary medical doctor may be an easier, and more realistic, first step toward the goal of confirming the disease.

Once confirmed, the F-A-C-S algorithm concludes with testing physical performance to determine severity. Physical performance not only involves the muscles, but also neurologic function and balance. For these reasons, these tests may not be possible to administer in people with dementia or those who have gait or balance disorders.

SARQOL QUESTIONNAIRE

The SarQoL Questionnaire, a self-assessment tool for people with confirmed sarcopenia, assesses the impact it has on their quality of life. It can identify potential problems and assess the impact of sarcopenia in all aspects of health. While still in its early days as a research tool, the SarQoL questionnaire is a valid tool to help health practitioners in understanding and addressing the challenges that sarcopenia creates. It is available for download at www. sarqol.org.

Severity

Gait Speed Test

One of the best ways to assess sarcopenia's severity is with the quick and easy gait speed test. In fact, how fast or slowly you move is so reliable at predicting the likelihood of falls, cognitive impairment, the need for institutionalization, and death, that this measurement has been referred to as the *sixth vital sign.* The test measures your usual walking speed; you may use an assistive device if necessary.

To Perform the Test:

1. On a flat unobstructed area, measure 4 meters (13 feet 1 inch), then mark the beginning and end with masking or painter's tape.

2. Stand 6 to 8 feet away from the starting line of tape and begin walking. This is in order to get you up to speed before you reach the start tape. You should have your phone on its stopwatch poised to hit start, or a watch with a second hand (or second display).

3. When the first foot to cross the starting line lands on the floor, hit start on your stopwatch (or glance at the second hand of your watch).

4. Stop the timer (or note the time) when the first foot to cross the finish line lands on the floor, but keep moving through the finish line so you don't prematurely decelerate.

Reference Range:

If it took you longer than 5 seconds to walk the 4 meters, you may have an increased risk of frailty and falls. Pursue a work-up for advanced sarcopenia and begin the treatment routines outlined in this book.

Short Physical Performance Battery

The Short Physical Performance Battery (SPPB), developed in 1994 by the National Institute on Aging (NIA), also measures the severity of sarcopenia. It consists of the gait speed test, a balance assessment, and the chair stand test. It is a relatively easy battery of tests to perform, has a cumulative point score system, and is an objective measure to evaluate lower extremity strength and function. It is available for use on the National Institute of Health's NIA website at www.nia.nih.gov/research/labs/leps/short-physical-performance-battery-sppb.

Afterword

Sarcopenia is quickly becoming one of the most significant and talked-about medical topics in years. Between the numerous and devastating health consequences of weakened and thinning muscles and the impressive ability of resistance training to reverse and prevent them, you can understand why.

Many mental and physical diseases that are taken for granted as the price of getting older do not have to be your destiny. Never has it been truer that exercise is medicine—medicine that is cheap, works fast, and significantly improves your health, fitness, confidence, and energy, with no negative side effects.

While many people remain active as they get older, you can be one of the select few who trains your body. What's the difference? Aside from all the previously discussed benefits, training is a rewarding activity that is goal-oriented, requires discipline, and creates a life with a mission to continually improve yourself. Make strength training an essential part of your fitness program and you won't have to find out what it's like to grow old without seeing the beauty and strength that your body is capable of, as Socrates admonished.

For questions, comments, and more information to help you on your path to maximal health, visit endeverydaypain.com.

To your health!

Notes

1.   Alex Han and Steven L. Bokshan, et al., "Diagnostic Criteria and Clinical Outcomes in Sarcopenia Research: A Literature Review," *Journal of Clinical Medicine* 7, no. 70 (2018).

2.   Alfonso J. Cruz-Jentoft and Gulistan Bahat, et al., "Sarcopenia: Revised European Consensus on Definition and Diagnosis," *Age and Aging* 48, no. 1 (2018): 1–16.

3.   Florida Atlantic University, "Skinny Fat in Older Adults May Predict Dementia, Alzheimer's Risk," *Science Daily (*July 5, 2018).

4.   Carla Coetsee and Elmarie Terblanche, "The Effect of Three Different Exercise Training Modalities on Cognitive Function in a Healthy Older Population," *European Review of Aging and Physical Activity* 14 (2017).

5.   Inhwan Lee and Jinkyung Cho, et al., "Sarcopenia Is Associated with Cognitive Impairment and Depression in Elderly Korean Women," *Iran Journal of Public Health* no. 3 (March 2018): 327–34.

6.   C. H. Wu and K. C. Yang, et al., "Sarcopenia Is Related to Increased Risk for Low Bone Mineral Density," *Journal of Clinical Densitometry* 16, no. 1 (January-March 2013): 98–103.

7.   Marlene Busko, "Sarcopenia May Signal Twofold Fracture in Healthy Elderly," *Medscape (*October 23, 2015), https://www.medscape.com/viewarticle/853150.

8.   T. Hida and N. Ishiguro, et al., "High Prevalence of Sarcopenia and Reduced Leg Muscle Mass in Japanese Patients Immediately After a Hip Fracture," *Geriatric Gerontology International* 13, no. 2 (April 2013): 413–20.

9.   Jorma Panula and Harri Pihlajamaki, et al., "Mortality and Cause of Death in Hip Fracture Patients Aged 65 or Older: A Population-Based Study," *BMC Musculoskeletal Disorders* 12 (May 2011): 105.

10. Jean-Yves Reginster and Charlotte Beaudart, et al., "Osteoporosis and Sarcopenia: Two Diseases or One?" *Current Opinion in Clinical Nutrition and Metabolic Care* 19, no. 1 (January 2016): 31–36.

11. Tetsuro Hida and Atushi Harada, et al., "Managing Sarcopenia and Its Related-Fractures to Improve Quality of Life in Geriatric Populations," *Aging and Disease* 5, no. 4 (August 2014): 226–37.

12. University of California, Los Angeles, Health Sciences, "Higher Muscle Mass Associated with Lower Mortality Risk in People with Heart Disease," *ScienceDaily*, April 26, 2016, accessed February 22, 2019, www .sciencedaily.com/releases/2016/04/160422080059.htm.

13. T. Hida and A. Harada, et al., "Managing Sarcopenia and Its Related-Fractures to Improve Quality of Life in Geriatric Populations," *Aging and Disease* 5, no. 4 (November 2013): 226–37.

14. Walter R. Frontera, Ana Rodriguez Zayas, and Natividad Rodriguez, "Aging of Human Muscle: Understanding Sarcopenia at the Single Muscle Cell Level," *Physical Medicine and Rehabilitation Clinics of North America* 23, no. 1 (February 2012): 201–207.

15. E. M. Strasser and M. Hofmann, "Strength Training Increases Skeletal Muscle Quality but Not Muscle Mass in Old Institutionalized Adults," *European Journal of Rehabilitation Medicine* 54, no. 6 (March 2018): 921–33.

16. J. B. Schoenfeld and B. Contreras, et al., "Resistance Training Volume Enhances Muscle Hypertrophy but Not Strength in Trained Men," *Medicine and Science in Sports and Exercise* 51, no. 1 (January 2019): 94–103.

17. M. Rondanelli and C. Klersy, et al., "Whey Protein, Amino Acids, and Vitamin D Supplementation with Physical Activity Increases Fat-Free Mass and Strength, Functionality, and Quality of Life and Decreases Inflammation in Sarcopenic Elderly," *America Journal of Clinical Nutrition* 13, no. 3 (March 2016): 830–40.

18. S. Basaria and A. D. Coviello, et al., "Adverse Events Associated with Testosterone Administration," *New England Journal of Medicine* 363, no. 2 (July 2010): 109–22

19. Tetsuharu Nakazono, Naoto Kamide, and Masataka Ando, "The Reference Values for Chair Stand Test in Healthy Japanese Older People: Determination by Meta-analysis," *Journal of Physical Therapy Science* 26, no. 11 (November 2014): 1729–31.

Bibliography

Basaria, S., and A. D. Coviello, et al. "Adverse Events Associated with Testosterone Administration." *New England Journal of Medicine* 363, no. 2 (July 2010): 109–22.

Bauer, Jurgen, and Gianni Biolo, et al. "Evidence-Based Recommendations for Optimal Protein Intake in Older People: A Position Paper from the PROT-AGE Study Group." *Journal of the American Medical Directors Association* 14 (2013): 542–59.

Busko, Marlene. "Sarcopenia May Signal Twofold Fracture in Healthy Elderly." October 23, 2015, https://www.medscape.com/viewarticle/853150.

Cawood, A. L., M. Elia, and R. J. Stratton. "Systematic Review and Meta-Analysis of the Effects of High Protein Oral Nutritional Supplements." *Ageing Research Reviews* 11, no. 2 (April 2012): 278–96.

Coetsee, Carla, and Elmarie Terblanche. "The Effect of Three Different Exercise Training Modalities on Cognitive Function in a Healthy Older Population." *European Review of Aging and Physical Activity,* 14 (2017).

Cosquéric, Gaëlle, and Aline Sebag, et al. "Sarcopenia Is Predictive of Nosocomial Infection in Care of the Elderly." *British Journal of Nutrition* 96, no. 5 (November 2006): 895–901.

Cruz-Jentoft, Alfonso J., and Gulistan Bahat, et al. "Sarcopenia: Revised European Consensus on Definition and Diagnosis." *Age and Ageing* 48, no. 1 (2018): 1–16.

Fiatarone, M. A., and E. F. O'Neill, et al. "Exercise Training and Nutritional Supplementation for Physical Frailty in Very Elderly People." *New England Journal of Medicine* 330, no. 25 (June 1994): 1769–75.

Florida Atlantic University. "Skinny Fat in Older Adults May Predict Dementia, Alzheimer's Risk." *Science Daily,* (July 5, 2018).

Forrest, K. Y., and W. L. Stuhldreher. "Prevalence and Correlates of Vitamin D Deficiency in US Adults." *Nutrition Research* 31, no. 1 (January 2011): 48–54.

Francis, Peter, and William McCormack, et al. "Twelve Weeks' Progressive Resistance Training Combines with Protein Supplementation Beyond Habitual Intake Increases Upper Leg Lean Tissue Mass, Muscle Strength and Extended Gait Speed in Healthy Older Women." *Biogerontology* 18, no. 6 (2017): 881–91.

Franzke, B., and O. Neubauer, D. Cameron-Smith, and K. H. Wagner. "Dietary Protein, Muscle and Physical Function in the Very Old." *Nutrients* 10, no. 7 (July 2018).

Frontera, Walter R., Ana Rodriguez Zayas, and Natividad Rodriguez. "Aging of Human Muscle: Understanding Sarcopenia at the Single Muscle Cell Level." *Physical Medicine and Rehabilitation Clinics of North America* 23, no. 1 (February 2012): 201–207.

Goldman, Tom. "Jack LaLanne: Founding Father of Fitness." *NPR*, January 24, 2011, https://www.npr.org/2011/01/24/133175583/jack-lalanne-founding-father-of-fitness.

Han, Alex, and Steven L. Bokshan, et al. "Diagnostic Criteria and Clinical Outcomes in Sarcopenia Research: A Literature Review." *Journal of Clinical Medicine* 7, no. 70 (2018).

Hida, Tetsuro, and Atushi Harada, et al. "Managing Sarcopenia and Its Related-Fractures to Improve Quality of Life in Geriatric Populations." *Aging and Disease* 5, no. 4 (August 2015) 226–37.

Hida Tetsuro, and Naoki Ishiguro, et al. "High Prevalence of Sarcopenia and Reduced Leg Muscle Mass in Japanese Patients Immediately After a Hip Fracture." *Geriatric Gerontology International* 13, no. 2 (April 2013): 413–20.

Jorgensen, P. B., and S. B. Bogh, et al. "The Efficacy of Early Initiated, Supervised, Progressive Resistance Training Compared to Unsupervised, Home-Based Exercise After Uncomplicated Knee Arthroplasty." *Clinical Rehabilitation* 31, no. 1 (January 2017): 61–70.

Kamen, Gary, and Christopher A. Knight. "Training-Related Adaptations in Motor Unit Discharge Rate in Young and Older Adults." *The Journals of Gerontology: Series A* 59, no. 12 (December 2004): 1334–38.

Lee, Bruce Y. "What Muscle Has to Do with Breast Cancer." Forbes.com, April 8, 2018, https://www.forbes.com/sites/brucelee/2018/04/08/what-muscle-has-to-do-with-breast-cancer-survival/#58b1a7221ada.

Lee, Inhwan, Jinkyung Cho, et al. "Sarcopenia Is Associated with Cognitive Impairment and Depression in Elderly Korean Women." *Iran Journal of Public Health* 47, no. 3 (March 2018): 327–34.

Malmstrom, T. K., and D. K. Miller et al. "SARC-F: A Symptom Score to Predict Persons with Sarcopenia at Risk for Poor Functional Outcomes." *Journal of Cachexia Sarcopenia Muscle* 7, no. 1 (March 2016): 28–36.

Miyakoshi, N. "Fall Risk Fracture. Vitamin D and Falls/Fractures." *Clinical Calcium* 23, no. 5 (May 2013): 695–700.

Nakazono, Tetsuharu, Naoto Kamide, and Masataka Ando. "The Reference Values for Chair Stand Test in Healthy Japanese Older People: Determination by Meta-Analysis." *Journal of Physical Therapy Science* 26, no. 11 (November 2014): 1729–31.

Nelson, M. E., and M. A. Fiatarone, et al. "Effects of High-Intensity Strength Training on Multiple Risk Factors for Osteoporotic Fractures. A Randomized Controlled Trial." *Journal of the American Medical Association* 272, no. 24, (December 1994): 1909–14.

Norton, C., and C. Toomey, et al. "Protein Supplementation at Breakfast and Lunch for 24 Weeks beyond Habitual Intake Increases Whole-Body Lean Tissue Mass in Healthy Older Adults." *The Journal of Nutrition* 146, no. 1 (January 2016): 65–69.

Panula, Jorma, and Harri Pihlajamaki, et al. "Mortality and Cause of Death in Hip Fracture Patients Aged 65 or Older: A Population-Based Study." *BMC Musculoskeletal Disorders* 12 (2011): 105.

Perkin, Oliver J., and Polly McGuigan, et al. "Habitual Physical Activity Levels Do Not Predict Leg Strength and Power in Healthy, Active Older Adults." *PLOS One* 13, no. 7 (July 2018).

Price, R. Kevin. "Cicero's Thoughts on Growing Older." *Successful Retirement Guide's Weblog,* December 6, 2009, http://successfulretirementguide.wordpress.com/2009/12/06.

Reginster, Jean-Yves, and Charlotte Beaudart, et al. "Osteoporosis and Sarcopenia: Two Diseases or One?" *Current Opinion in Clinical Nutrition and Metabolic Care* 19, no. 1 (January 2016): 31–36.

Rondanelli, M., and C. Klersy, et al. "Whey Protein, Amino Acids, and Vitamin D Supplementation with Physical Activity Increases Fat-Free Mass and Strength, Functionality, and Quality of Life and Decreases Inflammation in Sarcopenic Elderly." *America Journal of Clinical Nutrition* 103, no. 3 (March 2016): 830–40.

Schoenfeld, B. J., and B. Contreras, et al. "Resistance Training Volume Enhances Muscle Hypertrophy but Not Strength in Trained Men." *Medicine and Science in Sports and Exercise* 51, no. 1 (January 2019): 94–103.

Shao, Andrew, and Wayne W. Campbell, et al. "The Emerging Global Phenomenon of Sarcopenic Obesity: Role of Functional Foods; a Conference Report." *Journal of Functional Foods* 33 (2017): 244–50.

Singh, N. A., and S. Quine, et al. "Effects of High-Intensity Progressive Resistance Training and Targeted Multidisciplinary Treatment of Frailty on Mortality and Nursing Home Admissions After Hip Fracture," *Journal of the American Medical Directors Association* 13, no. 1 (January 2012): 24–30.

Siparsky, P. N., D. T. Kirkendall, and W. E. Garrett Jr. "Muscle Changes in Aging: Understanding Sarcopenia," *Sports Health* 6, no. 1 (January 2014): 36–40.

Strasser, E. M., and M. Hofmann, et al. "Strength Training Increases Skeletal Muscle Quality but Not Muscle Mass in Old Institutionalized Adults." *European Journal of Rehabilitation Medicine* 54, no. 6 (March 2018): 921–33.

Tieland, M., and O. van de Rest, et al. "Protein Supplementation Improves Physical Performance in Frail Elderly People: A Randomized, Double-Blind, Placebo-Controlled Trial." *Journal of American Medical Directors Association* 13, no. 8 (October 2012): 720–26.

Tolea, Magdalena, and James E. Galvin. "Sarcopenia and Impairment in Cognitive and Physical Performance," *Clinical Interventions in Aging* 10 (2015): 663–71.

University of California, Los Angeles, Health Sciences. "Higher Muscle Mass Associated with Lower Mortality Risk in People with Heart Disease." *ScienceDaily*, (April 26, 2016, accessed February 22, 2019), www.sciencedaily.com/releases/2016/04/160422080059.htm.

Wolfe, R. R. "The Role of Dietary Protein in Optimizing Muscle Mass, Function, and Health Outcomes in Older Individuals." *British Journal of Nutrition* 108, suppl. 2 (August 2012): 588–93.

Wu, C. H., and K. C. Yang, et al. "Sarcopenia Is Related to Increased Risk for Low Bone Mineral Density." *Journal of Clinical Densitometry* 16, no. 1 (January-March 2013): 98–103.

Yu, Jie. "The Etiology and Exercise Implications of Sarcopenia in the Elderly." *International Journal of Nursing Sciences* 2, no. 2 (June 2014): 199–203.

Index

Activities of daily living (ADLs), 17

Acute sarcopenia, 14–15

Aerobic exercise, 10; vs. strength training, 29; and warming up, 32; workouts (HIIT), 53

Alzheimer's disease, 18

American College of Sports Medicine (ACSM), 53

Amino acids, 101, 102, 105, 106–107; leucine, 110

Anabolism, 101, 102

Animal proteins, 105

Ankle weights, 58

Arm Circles, 33

Arm/shoulder exercises. *See* Upper-body exercises

Arm/shoulder: stretches, 33–35, 45

Assessment tests, for sarcopenia, 112–14

Back exercises. *See* Lower-body exercises; Upper-body exercises

Back (lower) Stretch, 46

Back of the Thigh Stretch, 49

Back stretches, 36–37, 46

Balance issues, and falls, 19; and PRE, 28–29; and vitamin D, 109

Bands, exercise, 58

Barbells, 58

Bent-Over Triceps Kick-Backs with Weights, 79

Biceps Curl with Resistance Tube, 78

Biceps Curl with Weights, 77

Bird Dog with Weights, 83

Bladder cancer, 22

Blood pressure. *See* Hypertension

Body fat, 15

Body weight, as exercise "equipment," 58

Bokshan, Steven L., quoted, 7

Bone disease/fractures, 19–20; and vitamin D, 109

Bone mineral density, 19

Breast cancer, 21

Breathing, and posture, 32

Calf Stretch, 50

Cancer, 21–22

Cardiovascular disease, 20–21; and omega-3s, 109

Casein protein, 107

Catabolism, 101

Causes, of sarcopenia, 15–17

Chair Squat with Resistance Tube, 93

Chair Squat with Weights, 92

Chair stand/rise test, 113

Chemotherapy, 21

Chest Fly with Resistance Tube, 73

Chest Fly with Weights, 72

Chest Press with Weights, 70

Cholesterol, 21

Chronic sarcopenia, 14–15

Cicero, Marcus Tullius, 8

Cirrhosis of the liver, 22

Cognitive disorders/impairments, 15, 18

Compound exercises, 55

Consequences, of sarcopenia, 17–23

Cooling down, 43; exercises, 44–51

Core: exercises, 81–86; stretches, 38–39

Curl-Up with Weights, 81

Curls (exercises): arm, 77–78; core, 81; legs, 90–91

Dementia, 18

Depression, 18

Diabetes, 20

Diet, 15, 25, 100–10; deficits, 100–102; and protein, 102–105; supplements, 106–10; tips, 106

Diseases: and protein, 102; and sarcopenia, 17–23. *See also specific diseases/health problems*

Dual-energy absorptiometry (DXA), 114

Dumbbells, 58

Dynamic stretches, 32–42; exercises, 33–42; arms/ shoulders, 33–35; back, 36–37; core, 38–39; lower body, 40–42

Egg albumin protein, 107

Elastic band resistance training, 27–28

Elderly: and PRE, 27–28; and protein (dietary), 100–102

Equipment, 58–59

EWGSOP (European Working Group on Sarcopenia in Older People), quoted, 13; and F-A-C-S process, 111–16; findings, 13–14

Executive function, 15

Exercise, and sarcopenia, 7–8, 9–10

Exercise bands, 58

Exercises, 60–99; compound vs. isolation, 55; core, 81–86; defined, 54–55; equipment, 58–59; frequency, 57; intensity, 55; lower body, 87–99; program, 52–59; repetitions, 56; rest, 57; safety issues, 30–31; sets, 56–57; stretches, 32–51; tips, 60–61; upper body, 62–80; variations, 57–58

F-A-C-S (Find-Assess-Confirm-Severity) process, 111–16; SARC-F questionnaire, 111–12; severity, 115–16; tests, 112–15

Falls. *See* Balance issues

Fat-frail (sarcopenic obesity), 15

Fitness plan, 52–59

Flexibility exercises, 43

Flys, 72–74

Foam-rolling, 43

Forced vital capacity, 21

Form, proper, 31–32

Fractures. *See* Bone disease/fractures

Frailty, and protein supplementation, 107–108

Free weights, 58

Frequency, of exercises, 57

Front of the Thigh Stretch, 48

Gait speed test, 115–16

Galvin, James, quoted, 18

Gear, 58–59

Glute Bridge, 38

Grip strength test, 112

Gym equipment, 59

Han, Alex, quoted, 7

Harada, Atushi, quoted, 24

HbA1c levels, 20

Heart problems, 20–21

Heel Raise with Resistance Tube, 99

Heel Raise with Weights, 98

Hida, Tetsuro, quoted, 24

High blood pressure. *See* Hypertension

Hip Stretch, 47

Hip Swings, 40

Homeostasis, 23

Hormones, 101

Hospitalization, and sarcopenia, 22

Hypertension, and cardiovascular disease, 20

Inchworm (stretch), 39

Inflammation, after exercise, 31

Inflammation, systemic, 15, 20; and diet, 106; and protein, 101

Insulin: resistance, 20; and omega-3s, 109; sensitivity, 17

Intensity, of exercises, 55

Isolation exercises, 55

Kettlebells, 58

Kidney disease, 22

Knee Circles, 42

Knee to Chest, 41

LaLanne, Jack, quoted, 12, 30

Lee, Bruce Y., quoted, 21

Leg exercises/stretches. *See* Lower-body

Leg extensions, 96–97

Leg Press with Resistance Tube, 89
Leg strength: and functional decline, 17; assessment, 112–14
Leucine, 110
Liver disease, 22
Log book, 59
Lower-Back Stretch, 46
Lower-body: exercises, 87–99; stretches, 40–42
Lower/upper back stretches, 36–47

Medicine balls, 58
Mediterranean diet, 106
Muscle fibrosis, 16
Muscle protein synthesis, 102
Muscles/muscle mass: challenging, 10, 24, 26; and disease, 19–22; and functional decline, 17; and protein (dietary), 102; and PRE, 25; and supplements, 107–108; and testosterone, 110; and thermoregulation, 23; and vitamin D, 109; and weight loss, 29

Neck Stretch, 44

Obesity, 15
Omega-3 supplements, 109
Osteoarthritis (OA), 87, 120
Osteopenia, 15, 19
Osteoporosis, 19–20; and PRE, 25–26; and sarcopenic obesity, 15; and vitamin D, 109
Osteosarcopenic obesity (OSO), 15
Overhead Press with Resistance Tube, 63
Overhead Press with Weights, 62

Pain, 31
Pancreatic cancer, 22
Plant-based proteins, 105
Posture, 32

PRE (progressive resistance exercise), 7–8, 10; defined, 54–55; and elderly, 27–28; and health, 27–28; exercises, 60–99; long-term benefits, 28–29; and muscles, 10; and osteoporosis, 25; program, 52–59; and protein, 102–103, 108; and strength/power, 26–27; as treatment, 24–29; and weight loss, 29
Prediabetes, 20
Presses: arms, 62–63; chest, 70–71; legs, 89
Primary sarcopenia, 14
Program, exercise, 52–59
Progressive resistance exercise. See PRE
Prone Extension with Weights, 84–86
Prone Leg Curl with Resistance Tube, 91
PROT-AGE study group, and protein recommendations, 102–103
Protein (dietary), 100–10; chart, 104–105; deficits, 100–102; recommendations, 102–105; supplements, 106–108; timing, 105; tips, 106; types, 105

Quad Setting, 87
Questionnaires, 111–12, 115

Renal cell cancer, 22
Repetitions, of exercises, 56
Resistance tubes/tubing, 58
Respiratory disease, 21
Rest days, 57
Reverse Fly with Weights, 74
Rows (exercise), 75–76

Safety issues, 30–31
Sandbags, 58
SARC-F questionnaire, 111–12
Sarcopenia, 7, 8, 13–14; causes, 15–17; classification, 13; consequences, 17–23; cost, 23; and diet, 100–10; and exercise, 7–8, 9–10; history, 8–9; patient experiences, 9; prevalence, 8; and protein (dietary), 100–105; self-tests, 111–16; supplements, 106–10; treatment, 24–29; types, 14–15

Sarcopenic obesity (SO), 15

SarQoL Questionnaire, 115

Seated Leg Extension with Resistance Tube, 97

Seated Leg Extension with Weights, 96

Seated Leg Raise with Weights, 88

Seated Row with Resistance Tube, 75

Secondary sarcopenia, 14

Sedentary lifestyle, 15, 20

Self-tests, for sarcopenia, 111–15

Sets, of exercises, 56–57

Severity, of sarcopenia, tests, 115–16

Shin Stretch, 51

Short Physical Performance Battery (SPPB), 116

Shoulder Blade Mobility (stretch), 35

Shoulder strengthening, 61

Shoulder Stretch, 45

Shoulder/arm exercises. *See* Upper-body exercises

Shoulder/arm stretches, 33–35, 45

Single-Arm Row with Weights, 76

Skeletal muscles, 15–16, 17; and cardiovascular disease, 21; and diabetes, 20

Skinny-fat (sarcopenic obesity), 15

SO (sarcopenic obesity), 15

Socrates, quoted, 60, 111

Soreness, 31

Speed (velocity), of exercises, 55

Squat with Resistance Tube, 95

Squat with Weights, 94

Squats, 92–95

Standing Chest Press with Resistance Tube, 71

Standing Leg Curl with Weights, 90

Standing Triceps Kick-Backs with Resistance Tubes, 80

Stanley, Edward, quoted, 52

Static stretches, 43–51; exercises, 44–51

Staying Young with Interval Training, 10, 26, 43, 57

Steroids, anabolic, 110

Stretches, 32–51; arms, 33–35; back, 36–37, 46; core, 38–39; dynamic, 32–42; lower body, 40–42; shoulder, 33–35, 45; static, 43–51

Supplements, dietary, 106–10

Tennis Backhand with Resistance Tube, 65

Tennis Backhand with Weights, 64

Tennis Forehand with Resistance Tube, 67

Tennis Forehand with Weights, 66

Testosterone, 110

Tests, for sarcopenia, 111–16

Thermoregulation, 23

Thigh exercises. See Lower-body exercises

Thigh stretches, 48–49

Thumbs Up with Resistance Tube, 69

Thumbs Up with Weights, 68

Timed chair stand test, 114

Timing, and protein intake, 105

Tolea, Magdalena, quoted, 18

Tools, 58–59

Treatment, of sarcopenia, 24–29

Trunk Rotation, 37

Trunk Rotation with Resistance Tube, 82

Trunk Side Bend, 36

Tubes/tubing, resistance, 58

Types, of sarcopenia, 14–15

Upper-body exercises, 62–80

Upper/lower back stretches, 36–37, 46

Variation, of exercise routine, 57–58

Vegetarians, 105, 106

Velocity, of exercises, 56

Vitamin D, as supplement, 109

Warming up, 32–42; exercises, 33–42

Weight machines, 59

Weight/weight loss, and PRE, 29

Weights, 58

Whey protein, 106; types, 107

Workout program, 52–59; intensity, 55

Wrist Circles, 34

Acknowledgments

A heartfelt thanks to Bridget Thoreson, acquisitions editor at Ulysses Press, for approaching me with this important and fascinating project. And to Casie Vogel, whom I suspect had something to do with it as well. To Claire Chun, for taking some technical writing and making it into a much more user-friendly story—thank you! And to Lily Chou, Lauren Harrison, and the rest of the team at Ulysses Press, for putting their faith in me to write yet another book, and then for working hard to make it a reality.

To two real American heroes, Andrew Taylor Still, DO, and Dr. William Garner Sutherland, DO, for being pioneers in their efforts to find health and not treat disease. To Dr. Jim Jealous, Dr. Jeff Greenfield, Dr. Hugh Ettlinger, and all the other osteopathic physicians who dropped breadcrumbs along the path less traveled, the healer's path. And to the thousands of patients and readers who put their faith in me to lead them to a healthier place—thank you.

And of course, a special thanks to my family. My wife, Janice, a true partner in life, parenthood, and camping. You're an amazing wife and mother—and nurse. Thanks for taking care of all of us. To my sweet not-so-little-anymore Lexi—thank you for playing office with me and writing your own book— "JJJKKKLMNN"—so that I could work on mine. And to littlest Madie, who occasionally parked in my lap while I wrote, here's to the first book of Daddy's you'll flip through without ripping or drooling on. Finally, to my mom, Patty; my mother-in-law, Debbie; and my father-in-law, Jim, thanks for all your help raising our girls!

About the Author

Dr. Joseph Tieri is an osteopathic physician and a specialist in the holistic hands-on healing practice of osteopathic manipulation. He is part owner and partner of the Stone Ridge Healing Arts Center and has been in private practice for 20 years. Dr. Tieri is also an associate professor at Touro College of Osteopathic Medicine, teaching the next generation of physicians the lost art of hands-on medicine.

Dr. Tieri is the author of *End Everyday Pain for 50+: A 10-Minute-a-Day Program of Stretching, Strengthening, and Movement to Break the Grip of Pain* and *Staying Young with Interval Training: The Revolutionary HIIT Approach to Getting Fit, Living Healthy and Keeping Muscles Young*.

For more information, please visit Endeverydaypain.com.